THE
EBOLA
SURVIVAL HANDBOOK

THE
EBOLA
SURVIVAL HANDBOOK

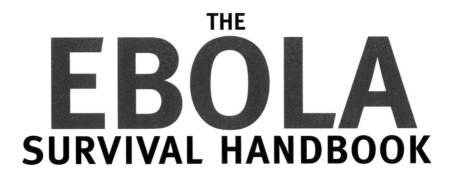

AN MD TELLS YOU WHAT YOU NEED TO KNOW NOW TO STAY SAFE

JOSEPH ALTON, MD

Skyhorse Publishing
New York

The information given in this volume is for educational and entertainment purposes only and does not constitute medical advice or the practice of medicine. No provider-patient relationship, explicit or implied, exists between the publisher, authors, and readers. This book does not substitute for such a relationship with a qualified provider. The strategies discussed in this volume are based on current knowledge; advances in our understanding of prevention, care, and treatment of Ebola virus may change significantly in the future. The authors and publisher strongly urge their readers to seek modern and standard medical care with certified practitioners whenever and wherever it is available.

The reader should never delay seeking medical advice, disregard medical advice, or discontinue medical treatment because of information in this book or any resources cited in this book.

Although the authors have researched all sources to ensure accuracy, they assume no responsibility for errors, omissions, or other inconsistencies therein. Neither do the authors or publisher assume liability for any harm caused by the use or misuse of any methods, products, instructions, or information in this book or any resources cited in this book.

Skyhorse Publishing books may be purchased in bulk at special discounts for sales promotion, corporate gifts, fund-raising, or educational purposes. Special editions can also be created to specifications. For details, contact the Special Sales Department, Skyhorse Publishing, 307 West 36th Street, 11th Floor, New York, NY 10018 or info@skyhorsepublishing.com.

Skyhorse® and Skyhorse Publishing® are registered trademarks of Skyhorse Publishing, Inc.®, a Delaware corporation.

Visit our website at www.skyhorsepublishing.com.

10 9 8 7 6 5 4 3 2 1

Library of Congress Cataloging-in-Publication Data is available on file.

Cover design by Brian Peterson
Cover photo by Thinkstock.com

Print ISBN: 978-1-63450-118-7
Ebook ISBN: 978-1-63450-119-4

Printed in the United States of America

This book is dedicated to nurses everywhere (including my lovely wife Amy who is a nurse). Nurses are the heart and soul of medical care, and even as a doctor, I could never achieve for a patient what they can do with a simple touch of their hand and a smile.

Author Bio

Joseph Alton, MD is a fellow of the American College of Surgeons and the American College of OB/GYN and the founder of the survival website DoomandBloom.net. Dr. Alton is the author of *The Survival Medicine Handbook* and is one of the most popular speakers in the country on crisis medicine. He has been featured in *The New York Times*, *Fortune* magazine, *The Miami Herald*, *Tulsa World*, *Small Business Trendsetters*, *Mother Jones*, and on various ABC, CBS, and Fox affiliates. Dr. Alton is a popular medical keynote speaker at survival and preparedness events throughout the country, and has been at the forefront of advising citizens on how to understand and survive the Ebola crisis.

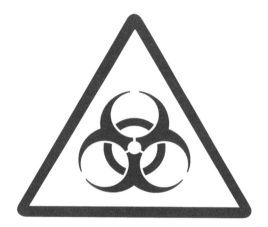

Contents

INTRODUCTION: An Unexpected Visitor

"TEXAS HEALTH WORKER TESTS POSITIVE FOR EBOLA"

That was the headline that greeted *Huffington Post* readers via email on a quiet Sunday morning.

This was big news. The medical system of a superpower nation had been trumped by a microscopic organism that looked like a strand of spaghetti. Ebola virus caused a major epidemic in a large region in Africa—all because someone ate bat meat that carried it.

By the end of the week, two nurses who treated Ebola patients in the United States had contracted the disease. These nurses, who were given minimal training in infectious-disease protocols, didn't just work behind the desk in the emergency room; they worked in an isolation area of an intensive care unit and wore protective gear.

But unlike cases before this, where the disease had been brought to the United States knowingly or unknowingly, these new developments made it clear that Ebola was no longer someone else's problem—it was now *our* problem.

The nurses did not contract Ebola deep in the jungle of some third-world country thousands of miles away but in a hospital in Texas. It infected a health-care worker, one of the people on the frontlines of disease control.

These represent the first known cases of transmission of the deadly virus in the United States, but will they be the last?

It's naïve to think so. The commissioner of the Texas Department of State Health Services, Dr. David Lakey, even admitted it in the *Huffington Post* when he stated, "We knew a second case could be a reality, and we've been preparing for this possibility. We are broadening our team in Dallas and working with extreme diligence to prevent further spread."

Ebola has become a reality to the average American. Of course, it doesn't always kill. Take the cases of the Americans who were treated, cured, and released back to their families. While their recovery may take a while, and they may never be at 100 percent (Dr. Sacra was readmitted for other reasons soon after his release), they are all still with us. The success has been attributed to good hospital care and access to an experimental drug that had not been previously tested on humans. Dr. Kent Brantley, a missionary with the North Carolina–based Samaritan's Purse who was evacuated from Liberia on August 2, 2014, said, "I am thrilled to be alive, to be well, and to be reunited with my family. As a medical missionary, I never imagined myself in this position."

I am also thrilled that Dr. Brantley is alive, but why are people dying from Ebola even though a serum exists that could save them? Why, in view of the dire situation in West Africa, are capable drugs being held back in a quagmire of government bureaucracy? And a bigger question is who decides who will get the drug and who won't?

It's not likely that your family doctor will be able to prescribe this medication anytime soon. I wrote this book because it's important to educate yourself about Ebola and prepare yourself for the small possibility of it coming to your neighborhood. There is no need for panic, but you, the average citizen, should take the time to learn about this deadly disease and how you can prevent it from affecting your family. It all starts with this book.

Ebola is real and the details can be frightening. The World Health Organization currently counts over ten thousand cases and five thousand deaths. If you're scared, you are not alone. According to a survey taken by Harris Poll/HealthDay, more than two thousand adults polled in the first week of October 2014 (a week before the death of the first US case), 27 percent viewed Ebola as a real threat to health and security. That figure was up from about 13 percent only weeks before. After Thomas Duncan's death, the numbers skyrocketed. By mid-October, about 55 percent polled believed Ebola was a serious health threat. People have cancelled holiday travel due to fear of Ebola. No infectious disease has generated this much concern since the HIV/AIDS pandemic.

Ebola is a "third-world disease" that is quickly becoming a "first-world disease." As Mayo Clinic's infectious diseases physician and researcher Dr. Pritish K. Tosh explains, "Ebola is an agent that evokes a lot of fear, and can result in societal disruption. There's a reason why it's considered a possible bioterrorism agent. So any time you have cases in the United States, there is a heightened amount of anxiety."

Bioterrorism is the weaponization of infectious germs and other agents to kill people and the animals and plants they depend on. Is Ebola a candidate for the next biological weapon? It has been rumored that Ebola is in inventory at high-level labs in many countries, some of which are not our friends.

We are assured that everything is under control. Western methods of taking care of the sick are more advanced; modern equipment is plentiful and available. Hospitals in the United States and other developed countries certainly have more resources than in the third-world countries, but mistakes have been made, and human error could be our downfall.

At the time of this book's publication, Ebola hemorrhagic fever kills at a 70 percent rate. While this is disturbing enough, the World Health Organization suggests that 1.4 million cases might be chronicled in the following few months.

How is this possible? As health-care workers contract Ebola from patients and bring it to their families, who bring it to people at work or school, who carry it home to *their* families—it begins a deadly cascade.

If we are complacent, we will see the numbers of American fatalities begin to shoot up. What can we do to prevent such a catastrophe? Of course, there are measures in place, but will enforcers strictly adhere to them? Have we done enough to prevent new cases from being imported from the Ebola zone? Ten thousand West Africans travel to the United States every three months through five major international airports:

- JFK International Airport in New York
- Washington Dulles International in Washington, DC
- O'Hare International in Chicago
- Hartsfield-Jackson International in Georgia
- Newark Liberty International in New Jersey

These airports now perform Ebola screenings for passengers who arrive from the three affected West African nations: Liberia, Sierra Leone, and Guinea. For more than 50 percent of Americans, however, a screening is not enough. The majority would prefer to see a total ban on allowing anyone traveling from those nations into the United States.

With that ban, Thomas Duncan would not have been allowed to come to the United States. He would not have infected the health-care workers who aided him, and this would have saved us millions of dollars in health-care costs and, more importantly, avoided putting American lives at risk.

There will inevitably be economic fallout if people keep getting sick. Hospitalization and treatment of just one Ebola patient takes up an incredible amount of resources. The World Bank recently estimated that, if the disease continued unabated, the economic impact of Ebola could reach $32.6 billion by the end of 2015. What could this mean for the rest of the world? The United States and Spain have already incurred significant costs evacuating their citizens in jets specially modified for infection control. The United States has committed to a large military presence in Liberia, ostensibly on humanitarian grounds. The expense is immense. Will Ebola bankrupt the United States by causing overwhelming financial and resource expenditures?

The bottom line is this: You can't depend on a pressured government to protect you against every sling and arrow that the uncertain future may hurl at you. Keeping yourself safe has to be in your hands. Luckily, it can be if you prepare yourself properly and take the proper precautions. With this guide, you will learn how to do just that.

I will provide a very specific understanding of the microbe that causes the disease, from its original appearance in the 1970s to the most recent epidemic. You'll get the nuts and bolts of how Ebola spreads in a way that is easy to understand. In this book you will find strategies that will help you stop Ebola from being transmitted to you and your loved ones. You will learn how to identify Ebola, with a complete list of signs and symptoms. I will outline how it gets diagnosed (or misdiagnosed) and how the illness is treated. You will know what the requirements are for treatment facilities and be able to assess whether or not your local hospital is prepared for an outbreak.

This guide details the ugly truth of what can happen when treatment fails. I will give notes on how to put together an effective sick room as well as the supplies necessary to deal with the sick. This will give you a plan of action and list of resources should Ebola ever expand to a worldwide pandemic.

In the past, Ebola may have seemed to be an issue that doesn't affect you or people you care about. That has changed. It's a serious health issue that could take you down in your own backyard at any time. Unless you arm yourself properly with skills, knowledge, and some basic supplies, you and your loved ones could face a future where this disease is not just a humanitarian concern, but a concern in your own home.

It's in your hands. Will you pick up the flag and get medically prepared? Someone has to. If you follow the advice in this book, you'll keep it together, even if everything else falls apart.

THE
EBOLA
SURVIVAL HANDBOOK

PART 1: WHAT IS YOUR RISK?

Once upon a time, in a land far, far away, Ebola was a disease that ravaged remote areas in the interior of the African continent. When Ebola moved closer to home, the days of no concern were over. The disease is now a global problem, and it pays to know more about it.

1. The History of Ebola—What Is It?

Ebola, also called Ebola hemorrhagic fever, is a disease that has a high fatality rate. The cause of Ebola is a virus that belongs to the Filoviridae family, most of which cause "hemorrhagic fevers." It can kill in several ways: internal bleeding, organ failure, and/or severe dehydration. When one contracts the disease, it will result in a massive viremia (large number of viruses in the blood) that damages the cells that form blood vessels. As the disease progresses, in some cases, uncontrolled bleeding leads to extreme fluid loss and can cause hypotensive shock. Most deaths, however, have occurred from organ failure and dehydration.

Ebola is "zoonotic," which means that it passes between animals and humans. The main reservoir is thought to be fruit bats, but it has been found in gorillas, monkeys, forest antelope, chimpanzees, and even porcupines.

Humans and apes can get the disease by coming into close contact with the body or bodily fluids (blood, vomit, mucus, droppings, etc.) of an infected animal. Other animals (say, an antelope) can get it by eating grass that has bat droppings on it.

Once the virus spreads to a human, person-to-person transmission is possible. It is highly contagious, with a mortality rate of between 50 and 95 percent, depending on the strain, promptness of treatment, level of medical resources available, and other factors.

The Ebola virus was initially discovered by an international team of scientists, including Dr. Peter Piot, Dr. Joel Breman, and researcher Karl Johnson. They were asked to look into the outbreak of a mysterious illness among villagers in Zaire, now the Democratic Republic of Congo. The first recorded case of Ebola was in 1976. A village schoolteacher had symptoms similar to those of malaria (a disease common in the region). The schoolteacher was treated with quinine, a drug commonly used on patients with malaria. However, the quinine did not clear up the problem. His condition worsened ,and he succumbed to the disease two weeks later. A number of people who cared for him developed the illness, and soon it spread to the entire village. This new virus had no name. The scientists tossed names around over a bottle of bourbon, and narrowed the choices down to the village in which they stayed and studied (Yambuku), or a nearby river, the Ebola. They chose Ebola as they didn't want the Yambuku villagers to be unfairly stigmatized.

GEOGRAPHICALLY NAMED VIRUSES

Ebola isn't the only disease that's been named after the region where it was discovered.

Bolivian Hemorrhagic Fever (a.k.a. Black Typhus, a.k.a. Machupo Virus)	An infectious disease caused by the Machupo virus that occurs in Bolivia and is transmitted through rodent droppings.
Coxsackievirus	Discovered in 1948 in Coxsackie, a town in New York, Coxsackie symptoms and signs include sore throat, rash, and blisters.
Hendra Virus	In 1944, Hendra virus was discovered following an outbreak of illness in horses in a large racing stable in the suburb of Hendra in Brisbane, Australia.
Marburg Virus	A hemorrhagic fever virus (similar to Ebola) discovered during small epidemics in the German cities Marburg and Frankfurt as well as in Yugoslav's capital, Belgrade, in 1967.
MERS-CoV	Middle East Respiratory Syndrome Coronavirus was first reported in 2012 after genome sequencing of a virus isolated from sputum samples in patients in twenty-two countries who had fallen in an outbreak of a new flu. However, all cases can be traced back to Saudi Arabia.

(Continued)

Ross River Virus	A virus named after a river in northern Queensland in Australia in 1937. It is an infection that causes major weakness in the body.
West Nile Virus	A virus transmitted by mosquitoes; most people infected may only experience fever and mild headache but others may develop a life-threatening illness that includes inflammation of the brain. It was first identified in the West Nile region of Uganda in 1937.

> **TIP**
>
> *There are currently five known strains of the ebola virus: Taï Forest, Sudan, Bundibugyo, Zaire, and Reston. All, with the exception of Reston, have been identified in humans.*

STRAINS OF EBOLA

There are currently five known varieties (also known as "strains") of the Ebola virus: Taï Forest, Sudan, Bundibugyo, Zaire, and Reston. All, with the exception of Reston, have been identified in humans.

TAÏ FOREST
Taï Forest (TAFV) virus was first identified as a new "strain" of Ebola virus in 1995 and has only had one known occurrence among humans, though it devastated the western chimpanzee population in Taï National Park, Côte d'Ivoire. While it is not known how TAFV infected these chimpanzees, bats are suspected.

SUDAN
This was identified in 1998 as Sudan Ebola virus and is endemic (a constant presence) in Sudan and Uganda.

BUNDIBUGYO
Bundibugyo (BDBV) was first discovered in August 2007 when an outbreak occurred in the Bundibugyo township in western

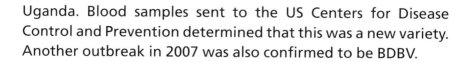

Uganda. Blood samples sent to the US Centers for Disease Control and Prevention determined that this was a new variety. Another outbreak in 2007 was also confirmed to be BDBV.

ZAIRE

Zaire is the most lethal of all Ebola strains. Endemic in Central Africa since 1976, it is the strain of the virus that is of the most concern throughout the world. It is thought to be the strain that has caused the current 2014 outbreak in West Africa.

RESTON

Reston virus (RESTV), named for Reston, Virginia, where the strain was first isolated in 1990, is a mutation from the Ebola virus discovered in a species of monkey imported from the Philippines. Reston virus is lethal to animals but has not, as yet, affected humans.

TIP

A special protein has been found to be essential both to the entry of Ebola and its replication. In laboratory tests, human cells that didn't have this transporter appeared impervious to Ebola when exposed. This suggests that some humans could be naturally resistant to the virus.

DOWN TO A SCIENCE

Understanding Ebola on a molecular level is the only way for researchers to figure out how it transmits to human cells and to develop new treatment methods and drugs that will stop it.

Scientifically speaking, Ebola virus observed under a microscope appears as a tubular strand approximately 80 nm in diameter and from 800 nm to 1,000 nm long. The overall shape varies, with only a few showing as simple cylinders while most exhibit branches, loops, coils, or hooks.

Like other viruses, Ebola is not by itself infectious. It requires a host cell (you!) to reproduce. This is different from bacteria, which can replicate on their own.

The virus penetrates the cell by attaching to certain receptors on the host. The viral membrane (or lining) fuses with the cell membrane. This releases its contents into the host. From there, the virus uses the cell's own corrupted internal mechanisms against it, eventually leading the cell to destroy itself.

A special protein has been found to be essential both to the entry of Ebola and its replication. In laboratory tests, human cells that didn't have this transporter appeared impervious to Ebola when exposed. This suggests that some humans could be naturally resistant to the virus.

ESSENTIAL EBOLA FACTS

* Ebola hemorrhagic fever is a disease caused by different strains of a virus first identified in the interior of Africa.

* Ebola infects various animals but seems to kill only humans and non-human primates, like chimpanzees.

* Ebola has, until recently, been contained in Africa. The current outbreak has a 70% death rate.

* Ebola has an incubation period (a period where you are infected but show no symptoms) of two to twenty-one days.

* Early Ebola symptoms can be confused with other infections at first, including influenza or malaria.

* Early symptoms of Ebola include: fever, headache, joint and muscle aches, sore throat, and weakness. Later symptoms include diarrhea, vomiting, stomach pain, hiccups, rashes, bleeding, and organ failure. When Ebola progresses to external and internal bleeding, it is almost always fatal.

* Ebola is most commonly spread by contact with blood and secretions, either via direct contact with the infected individual or fluids on clothing or other surfaces, as well as needles.

* At the highest risk for Ebola are those who live or travel to infected regions and have come in close contact with an infected person.

* The disease remains transmissible for a time in patients and in certain body fluids (such as semen) of those who recover.

* At present, there is no FDA-approved treatment for Ebola, although some promising drugs and vaccines are being developed and tested.

TIP

Early symptoms of Ebola include: fever, headache, joint and muscle aches, sore throat, and weakness. Later symptoms include diarrhea, vomiting, stomach pain, hiccups, rashes, bleeding, and organ failure. When Ebola progresses to external and internal bleeding, it is almost always fatal.

These tests are bringing scientists closer to a method of stopping the viral replication of Ebola, but they are not there yet. Experimental drugs and serums have been created that derived from this research, but these have not been fully tested. The process for approval of a new treatment or medication, at least in the United States, is often a slow and arduous one. The hope is that there is still time for science to win the race against the spread of the disease.

NOW YOU KNOW . . .
Ebola is a deadly virus that attacks healthy cells and replicates itself in a host's body. It is commonly, but not always, fatal. Discovered in 1976 in Central Africa, the current outbreak is in the more heavily populated countries of West Africa. Promising treatments and vaccines are in development and being tested, but are not yet officially approved by the Food and Drug Administration.

2. How Does Ebola Spread?

If Ebola has been contained in West Africa for nearly forty years, how is it, all of a sudden, a concern for the West? One reason is that the countries affected by the current outbreak are more heavily populated than previous outbreaks. With unrestricted commercial air travel, infectious organisms can spread faster than ever before.

Ebola also spreads when the proper precautions to contain it are not taken. Even when the correct procedures are adhered to, human error is an issue. In October 2014, the theoretical spread of Ebola into the western hemisphere became very real when Thomas Duncan entered the United States from Liberia. He was already infected with Ebola and started developing symptoms within a few days. Yet, due to a failure in the chain of communication, he was misdiagnosed with influenza and released back into the public. For the next two days, the highly contagious Mr. Duncan came into contact with one hundred other people before returning to the hospital in an ambulance.

Let's follow his journey from Liberia. Imagine all the ticket takers, fellow passengers, flight crews, airport personnel at his destination, the driver who took him to the place he was staying, the people he visited. What if Mr. Duncan had gotten a paper cut from his boarding pass? What if he got motion sickness in a cab and vomited in the back seat? Either of these scenarios, and others, could have happened. It is certainly known that he vomited outside the apartment where he was staying.

If just a few people had been infected, the ever-widening circle of contacts would have been tremendous. End result? An epidemic in the United States.

The previous situation with Ebola was that it would devastate some sparsely populated areas with a lack of resources and then eventually burn out. It was out of control in isolated small villages, but soon those that would die did, and the survivors either stayed or moved away once they recovered.

Extreme poverty and lack of resources are a contributing factor to the spread of Ebola. However, it goes well beyond financial or educational deficits. Consider this scary scenario that was recently reported by the World Health Organization: "In Sierra Leone, bodies of Ebola victims have been left in the street because of a strike by burial teams, who complain they have not been paid." Remember that Ebola is not just contagious from being in contact with a living victim; it remains contagious even after the victim has died. Picking up a discarded towel that had been used in the treatment of an Ebola victim and is encrusted with blood and other fluids creates just as lethal a risk. Imagine infected corpses lining the streets where people walk and commerce occurs and you can see the full extent of the problem.

In March 2014, infected persons from smaller towns began to be moved to larger hospitals in major cities. This has only created larger issues. There are too many patients and not enough hospital beds or health-care workers. At one point, there were one thousand Ebola patients in Monrovia, the capital of Liberia, and only 240 hospital beds for them. There are two doctors per 100,000 people in Sierra Leone, compared with 2.5 per 1,000 people in the United States. Some of the few doctors available were the first to contract the virus and die.

TIP

Remember that Ebola is not just contagious from being in contact with a living victim; it remains contagious even after the victim has died.

So, as time goes on, the situation worsens. It hasn't helped that the global community is coming in a day late and a dollar short. A condition that was once contained in the farthest reaches of the world has decimated several African countries' populations and economies and made its way to Europe and the United States.

FROM ANIMALS TO HUMANS

Ebola is not the only malady known to derive from interspecies contact. Scientists have estimated that six to ten of all infectious diseases in humans are spread from animals. Whether from a bite or other contact, humans have contracted a number of serious diseases from animals.

Bubonic Plague	Also known as the "Black Death," the Bubonic plague took down more than a quarter of the population of Europe and Asia in the fourteenth century. The bacterial disease has symptoms including fever, chills, weakness, and swollen and painful lymph nodes, and is carried by fleas on rodents and sometimes cats.
Chagas Disease	A frequently fatal infection transmitted by the feces of blood-feeding bugs called triatomines, which may live on dogs, chickens, or other domesticated animals.
HIV	HIV, short for human immunodeficiency, is the virus that causes AIDS. It kills by destroying the human immune system and has been traced back a century from contact with chimps and other primates. HIV was first documented in the United States in 1981.
Hantavirus	Hantavirus, carried mostly by deer mice, is contracted by breathing in dust contaminated with mouse droppings. Symptoms include a stiff neck, fever, and confusion. It's incurable but is generally not fatal.

Malaria	Spread by mosquitoes and most prominently found in hot, humid climates, malaria infects 350 million or more people every year.
Rabies	While infected dogs are mainly responsible for transmitting this disease by biting humans, many wild animals can carry rabies, including bats.
Influenza	Various types of flu viruses begin with an animal "reservoir." For example, H1N1 (swine flu) began with pigs, and bird flu started with domesticated poultry.
Toxoplasmosis	The toxoplasma gondii parasite infects about fifty million Americans, and its primary host is house cats. Transmission to humans is through cat feces, which is why pregnant women are warned against changing litter boxes.

THE SPREAD OF EBOLA

Ebola has been around since 1976, but not as an ongoing condition. While the disease has never been eradicated, outbreaks seem to go into periods of growth and, for want of a better term, "remission." Sometimes years will go by between outbreaks of the deadly disease, which sparks curiosity about how it continues even when it seems dormant for periods of time.

There are several methods of transmission of the Ebola virus. Here's how you can and can't get the virus, at least from our current knowledge.

Ingestion—Eating infected animals, especially if undercooked. This is the most likely way that Ebola began in the human population of West Africa, where infected bats are part of the diet.

You cannot get Ebola, however, from simply eating food at the same table as someone who has it or drinking from a water source in an area that has Ebola patients.

Inhalation—Breathing in droplets of blood splatter, vomit, or saliva of an infected patient. It is unlikely you will get it by simply breathing the same air in the room as someone who has it, although new commentaries from the Center of Infectious Disease Research and Policy (CIDRAP) and the US Army Medical Research Institute of Infectious Diseases (USAMRIID) are casting doubt on this. CIDRAP suggests that previously unexpected smaller viral particles may stay in the air in aerosol form. If this is the case, these particles may stay suspended for more than ninety minutes.

TIP

You cannot get Ebola from simply eating food at the same table as someone who has it or drinking from a water source in an area that has Ebola patients.

Another argument for airborne transmission comes from a 2012 study in which pigs were infected with Ebola virus in the same room as monkeys (separated by three meters). The monkeys contracted the virus without any known contact with the pigs.

The question of whether Ebola is "airborne" may be a matter of semantics. You could get Ebola if, for example, blood splatter is flung into the air and lands in your eye or nose. Certainly, this can be considered "airborne," but a better term would be "aerosol transmissible," in this case, with blood droplets.

Injection—Handling contaminated needles, syringes, or other medical supplies used on an infected individual. "Injection" could possibly include a bite from an animal carrying the Ebola virus. Dogs can be infected with Ebola without any noticeable effects but might be able to pass the virus to a human they bite. In fact, it is thought that 9–25 percent of all dogs in the epidemic zone carry the antibody for the virus. This means that there is evidence that they were, at one point, infected.

Absorption—Touching secretions from an infected individual and then touching your mouth or an open sore.

Sexual transmission—Ebola can be transmitted through sexual contact with someone who is infected. Interestingly, the semen of an infected individual is contagious for up to two months even if they have recovered from the illness.

Pregnancy—The virus may be passed from mother to fetus, even during breastfeeding.

Complacency—Complacency in our attitude toward infection control precautions may be the ultimate downfall when it comes to transmission of Ebola. If we do not pay strict attention to hand washing and other hygienic measures, we may pay the price.

Could Ebola mutate to the point that it will become absolutely airborne like influenza? Most experts say no; as so far it hasn't been the case with any strain of the virus. Also, as there has been so little change in the virus in the past forty years, it's unlikely that it would suddenly take on new and insidious characteristics.

Ebola spreads easily when the right care isn't taken in its treatment or when it isn't diagnosed correctly. When precautions are taken and care employed from the first sign of fever, it is actually fairly simple to contain. This is why it's important to know right away what health-care workers are dealing with—a painful lesson for us recently in the United States and also in Spain.

TIP

Ebola spreads easily when the right care isn't taken in its treatment or when it isn't diagnosed correctly. When precautions are taken and care employed from the first sign of fever, it is actually fairly simple to contain.

EBOLA IN SPAIN

In September 2014, Teresa Romero, an assistant nurse in Madrid, Spain, was infected with the Ebola virus after caring for a Spanish missionary who had been sent home from Liberia with the disease. The missionary (and a second one) succumbed to the illness. Ms. Romero had apparently gone undiagnosed for days, despite that she had: 1) been treating two patients with Ebola, and 2) developed a fever.

Health officials suspect that she may have inadvertently touched her face with a gloved hand—a quick, thoughtless gesture that could have happened to anyone. It was that simple. Human error again plays a part.

The patient, Manuel García Viejo, who had been medical director of a Sierra Leone hospital for twelve years, passed away from Ebola on September 25, 2014. Another nurse who had aided in his care was tested several times and finally released from the hospital after all tests for Ebola came back negative. At the time of this writing, Ms. Romero is still hospitalized. Her dog was euthanized.

Madrid is not the Third World. How could this happen in a first-world hospital? An investigation by the European Center for Disease Prevention and Control determined that despite the advancements the hospital had to offer, it lacked the proper capacity to handle emergencies such as an Ebola outbreak. The Health Ministry's coordinator of emergency alerts, Fernando Simón, reported, "The airlocks were set up to deal with highly infectious situations, but what hadn't been foreseen was a need for bulky outfits to perform certain medical procedures in."

We'll look at how to find out if your hospital is equipped to deal with an Ebola outbreak later in this book, but as you can see, even in the best, most secure hospitals, human error will always be an issue.

EBOLA SPREADS TO THE UNITED STATES

There was an uproar when confirmed American Ebola victims Dr. Kent Brantley and Nancy Writebol were transported to Emory Hospital in Atlanta, Georgia, from Liberia in the late summer of 2014. Ebola had not touched America in this way before—it had always been something contained on a continent hundreds of miles from home.

Emory Hospital proved to be an effective container for the disease. Neither Brantley or Writebol contaminated any of the medical staff, and in a matter of weeks, both recovered and

TIP

Patients who survive the virus receive, at least for ten years, immunity from the same Ebola strain.

were sent home with no trace of it remaining. Indeed, patients who survive the virus receive, at least for ten years, immunity from the same Ebola strain.

Texas Health Presbyterian Hospital in Dallas, however, did not have the same resources and capabilities. When Thomas Duncan first came to the hospital, he was sent home with antibiotics despite having a fever of 103 degrees and admitting to his recent arrival from the Ebola zone. At this point, he had already been incubating the disease for several days. Two days later, he returned to the hospital where he was diagnosed with Ebola on September 28, 2014, but by October 8 he was dead.

Thomas Duncan was a courier service driver in Liberia's capital, Monrovia. He had traveled to the United States to visit his former girlfriend and their nineteen-year-old son. Shortly before he left West Africa, Mr. Duncan had taken Marthalene Williams, a young Ebola patient, to a hospital where she was turned away due to lack of space. He then helped carry her home. Ms. Williams died of Ebola several hours later in his presence. As an aside, her brother, who had also helped carry her to and from the hospital, died from Ebola several days later.

A statement from the hospital's administration said, "We have made changes to our intake process as well as other procedures to better screen for all critical indicators of Ebola virus." However, the failure of the hospital was multifold. It should have demanded an immediate transfer of Mr. Duncan to one of the four high-risk infectious disease centers in the United States instead of handling the case itself. It should have instituted a rigorous training program to educate the nurses and other staff. The first two days of Mr. Duncan's admission, nurses wore wearing little protective gear while performing their duties. It is rumored that infected waste like bedding was piled to the ceiling of the hospital room.

What will be the fate of the people who cared for the medical staff stricken with the deadly virus? Ebola has been particularly cruel to heath-care workers, with hundreds in West Africa contracting and dying from the disease.

THE CHOCOLATE FACTOR

You know that Ebola is a serious health threat, but it also poses economic threats beyond the cost of health-care and military expenses. The economies of some countries in West Africa have come to a standstill due to Ebola. A huge industry that affects the average American is also being hurt by restrictions tied to areas deeply affected by Ebola: The chocolate industry. According to a recent article on Politico.com:

> The countries with the worst Ebola outbreaks neighbor three countries that produce almost 60 percent of the world's chocolate production. "Prices on cocoa futures jumped from their normal trading range of $2,000 to $2,700 per ton, to as high as $3,400 over concerns about the spread of Ebola to Côte D'Ivoire (French for Ivory Coast)," noted Jack Scoville, an analyst and vice president at the Chicago-based Price Futures Group. "Since then, prices have yo-yoed down to $3,030 and then back to $3,155 in the past couple of weeks."

The Ivory Coast, a small nation that borders both Liberia and Guinea, produces more than 33 percent of the world's total cocoa beans. As a result of the epidemic, it has closed its borders. A large portion of the work force needed to harvest the cocoa beans (that eventually become chocolate) come from the neighboring countries. This will likely mean an increase in the cost of cocoa beans, and therefore, a spike in the cost of chocolate. From the same article, "The World Cocoa Foundation is working now to collect large donations from Nestlé, Mars, and 113 other members for its Cocoa Industry Response to Ebola Initiative." The Ebola epidemic, even in far-away West Africa, affects us all in many ways.

NOW YOU KNOW . . .

So now you know the various ways that you can get Ebola, and how you can't. It isn't the easiest virus to get but that doesn't mean it's impossible either. All it takes is our continued failure to take the measures necessary to protect our health-care workers and our failure to restrict travel from the epidemic zone. Now, would you recognize an Ebola victim if you saw one? Keep reading to learn how.

3. Signs & Symptoms

In all that we've learned in the past decades about Ebola, one of the most effective ways to ensure survival is to treat the disease immediately. When symptoms arise, it's important to keep in the back of one's mind that what might seem like a simple bout of the flu could very well turn out to be Ebola. Once the later symptoms of the disease begin to present themselves, it is almost always too late.

In this chapter, we'll break down the signs and symptoms that very well could indicate an Ebola infection. Don't be dismissive if you begin to show any of these symptoms. It is probably something else, maybe the flu, but those who seek help early for either the flu or Ebola will be in better shape than those who don't.

NANCY'S "MALARIA"

Nancy Writebol was working with the missionary group Serving In Mission (SIM), an international organization with more than 1,600 active missionaries serving in more than sixty countries. Her job was to ensure that doctors working with Ebola patients were suited up properly in their personal protective gear. The tragic irony here is that she herself had not been properly protected. Ms. Writebol contracted Ebola and had to eventually be evacuated from Liberia. At first, however, it wasn't clear that she had contracted Ebola, despite the nature of the service she was performing. Even people working deep in the trenches of the epicenter of the outbreak often believe that their symptoms are not caused by Ebola. In all fairness, malaria is much more common than Ebola, and kills many more people. It is common that most people with symptoms of Ebola just assumed it was an episode of the ubiquitous mosquito-borne illness.

In any case, Ms. Writebol did not think she had Ebola. True, she wasn't feeling well and she had a fever, but she assumed it was malaria. "I had had malaria once in this past year, and so I knew what that felt like. And it was just the same symptoms," said Writebol.

If you tell a health-care provider that you've traveled from Africa and you're exhibiting a fever, that provider might easily be led to believe that you suffer from malaria. Indeed, the majority of suspected Ebola cases in the United States turn out to be malaria or some other illness.

Everyone, including Nancy, assumed that malaria was what ailed her, and could have very well treated her with quinine, but thankfully, they were vigilant. They decided to cover their bases, and they tested her for Ebola, even though she had previously been diagnosed with malaria. This high index of suspicion saved her life.

Ms. Writebol was immediately isolated and given ZMapp, an experimental Ebola drug that had, at that point, only been tested on monkeys. She was then evacuated for treatment in the United States. It was because of the swift diagnosis and treatment that she recovered.

While Ebola vaccines are still in human trials, experimental treatments like ZMapp have been showing favorable results. When you ignore the signs and symptoms of Ebola, you put not only yourself but everyone you come in contact with at high risk.

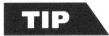

After a period of 2–21 days (average 8–10) without symptoms, the Ebola patient begins to show signs of the disease.

WHAT YOU NEED TO LOOK OUT FOR . . .

After a period of 2–21 days (average 8–10) without symptoms, the Ebola patient begins to show signs of the disease. The signs and symptoms of Ebola can be divided into early, middle, and late stages.

EARLY STAGES

In the early stages of Ebola, it looks like a lot of other illnesses. You might notice:

- Aches and pains
- Cough
- Sore throat
- Shortness of breath
- Fever and chills
- Headache
- Nausea
- Hiccups
- A general ill feeling (otherwise known as malaise)

Other than hiccups, which occur only in a percentage of cases, this sounds like the flu, doesn't it?

MIDDLE STAGES
As the disease progresses, you might see:

- Rashes
- Eye redness (similar to pinkeye or conjunctivitis)
- Vomiting
- Diarrhea

LATE STAGES
Once the disease progresses to the later stages, the patient is in bad shape. Signs and symptoms include:

- Altered mental status
- Seizures
- Difficulty breathing
- Dark red coloration of the roof of the mouth
- Bruises
- Broken blood vessels in the skin
- Collections of blood under the skin after injections
- Bloody vomit or sputum
- Spontaneous nosebleeds
- Bleeding from gums
- Blood in bowel movements

It should be noted that, although Ebola is classified as a hemorrhagic fever, only about 50 percent of victims show evidence of abnormal bleeding. Patients will show a subset of the above signs and symptoms; in other words, they will show some of them and not show others.

Although the classic case has major bleeding issues, the most common cause of death is multiple organ failures and severe dehydration.

LAB FINDINGS

The symptoms are how Ebola manifests outwardly, but the disease does incredible damage to your overall body chemistry. This is reflected in various lab tests, most results of which can be available in a relatively short time (if the lab has the proper equipment).

The information received from laboratory findings aids physicians in determining how much overall damage Ebola has caused in patients, and alerts them to other conditions that may arise as a result of the infection. We'll get more into the "aftereffects" of Ebola in the next chapter.

NOW YOU KNOW . . .

The symptoms of Ebola are very similar to the flu and malaria. Because the signs and symptoms are similar, Ebola can go undiagnosed, which creates a number of issues. This increases the possibility of Ebola spreading to anyone the patient may come in contact with after being misdiagnosed. If someone seems to exhibit any of the symptoms of Ebola, it is essential that they be tested and receive medical attention as soon as possible.

4. Diagnosis & Treatment

Now that Ebola has infiltrated our national health infrastructure, it is important not to instantly panic and believe you have contracted Ebola because you live in Atlanta or Dallas or that you recently sat with a friendly Liberian on an airplane. Panic is as bad as complacency when it comes to epidemics.

Yes, keep aware of the signs. Keep vigilant about washing your hands and pay attention to people you encounter over the course of your day. And if you have any doubts at all, please see your doctor.

Ebola can only be diagnosed by a physician after tests have been done on your blood, urine, and so forth. The CDC is working to ensure that health-care professionals run these tests on anyone who might seem suspect.

Be mindful, however, that you will be told that not everyone who comes into hospitals exhibiting symptoms similar to those of Ebola will be tested for Ebola. Remember that the signs and symptoms of the disease are similar to so many other diseases, especially in the first week of having those symptoms. There have been many cases of people being tested for Ebola who end up not having the disease. Recently, a pair was taken to New York's Bellevue Hospital as they were exhibiting signs of illness. In the last two months, Bellevue alone has handled at least twenty-nine suspected cases of Ebola. None of the patients actually had the deadly virus. The official statement made by Bellevue hospital reads:

> There are no patients at Bellevue with Ebola. Two patients there this morning were evaluated and it was quickly determined they did not have the virus. Because of the heightened alert, hospitals will be using enhanced scrutiny and

an abundance of caution when reviewing questionable cases, and are meticulously following all public health and CDC protocols.

If you have reason to believe you could have Ebola, it's crucial that you bring those reasons with you to your examination, including travel documentation or any evidence you may have that may connect you to a person known to have contracted Ebola. Without a convincing argument, it's possible you won't be tested for Ebola. Hospitals will claim they simply don't have the resources to test everyone for the disease. Be sure to go to the hospital or doctor's office prepared to state your case.

DIAGNOSING EBOLA

The thing is, chances are pretty good that your doctor will not test you for Ebola unless you have come in contact with someone who has Ebola, or someone who has come in contact with someone who has Ebola and then come in contact with you. If you feel sick or have a fever after coming in contact with someone recently arrived from a region of Ebola outbreak or a hospital worker treating Ebola, it is important to bring this information to your doctor's attention.

In the first few days after symptoms develop, you will be tested for Ebola if there is adequate reason to believe you are at risk. There are special tests which are sent to the CDC and analyzed within a twenty-four to forty-eight hour period.

TIP

If you feel sick or have a fever after coming in contact with someone recently arrived from a region of Ebola outbreak or a hospital worker treating Ebola, it is important to bring this information to your doctor's attention.

If you are diagnosed with Ebola after the results from these tests come back, you will be hospitalized (hopefully in a high-risk center). Once you have recovered, you will likely be given additional testing to detect for "antibodies." These are certain Y-shaped proteins that your body produces to deactivate dangerous viruses and bacteria. Some of the tests include:

ELISA
If you are infected and have survived long enough to begin developing immunity, Enzyme Linked Immunosorbent Assay (ELISA) tests can be useful in detecting Ebola. There are two varieties, immunoglobulin M (IgM) and immunoglobulin G (IgG), and both can show specific and accurate results.

PCR
This test (officially known as "reverse transcriptase polymerase chain reaction" or PCR) is used to detect genetic material from the virus and can pick up very small quantities. That means it could be a good tool for early detection but that it can come back falsely negative during the first three days of infection.

VIRUS ISOLATION

Virus isolation can be effective but can be dangerous and should only be done in lab with high-level biosafety (level 4) conditions firmly in place. Due to the inherent risks involved in culturing and replicating Ebola, even in a controlled environment, this type of test is more difficult to perform. Instead of being used to examine the situation of one patient, it can be used in research to better understand Ebola, leading to effective treatment drugs and, eventually, a vaccine.

Various other tests that determine the state of your blood, especially clotting factors, and the function of various organs will be performed.

TREATING EBOLA

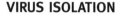

There is no cure for Ebola as of the time of this writing. However, patients have been documented to make full recoveries based solely on "supportive therapy," which encompasses measures taken to balance fluids and electrolytes, maintaining oxygen status and blood pressure, and working to avoid any complicating infections. It is well documented that patients who are hospitalized, in general, do better than those in West Africa that are turned away due to lack of bed space. Even the prevention of dehydration with simple IV fluids may improve the chance of recovery.

The Food and Drug Administration (FDA) has not yet officially approved a drug or vaccine as effective against the Ebola virus. However, there are a number of very promising agents that will, hopefully, be available soon. Even so, the question of how fast large quantities can be manufactured exists. And if there are limited amounts of vaccine or treatment, who gets it and who doesn't?

ZMAPP

The treatment receiving the most attention is called "ZMapp." ZMapp has been credited with aiding the recovery of several missionaries evacuated to the United States after being infected in West Africa.

ZMapp therapy consists of three "monoclonal antibodies" that are designed to treat existing Ebola infection. These antibodies work by binding to proteins in the virus and "targeting" them for destruction by the immune system.

To explain simply how ZMapp is made, a mouse is injected with Ebola. It produces antibodies against the viruses, which are taken and combined with human cells. Now you have cells with genetic material from two species (called a "chimera" after a mythological beast made up of parts of different animals). These cells, theoretically, have the capacity to fight the virus. They are cloned to make a serum that is given to Ebola victims. It's more complex than this, but this is an easy, simple description. Interestingly, the process uses tobacco plant material in production.

The serum has been successful in monkeys and may have been a factor in the recovery of some of the test subjects. The question being asked, however, is did the patients recover due to ZMapp, or was it due to their evacuation to high-level medical facilities or some genetic resistance to the virus?

Other drugs such as Tekmira are also in development in the FDA pipeline.

SURVIVOR BLOOD

There's also a growing movement to use whole blood or plasma from recovered Ebola patients in the treatment of Ebola sufferers. These survivors have antibodies which have successfully fought the virus. It is not proven to be effective, but is promising enough that it has spawned a burgeoning black market in Ebola survivor blood in West Africa.

AN EBOLA VACCINE?

While an FDA-approved Ebola vaccine isn't yet available, The National Institute of Allergy and Infectious Disease (NIAID), a division of the National Institutes of Health (NIH), is currently evaluating two candidates under serious consideration. A statement from the WHO on September 2, 2014, after a summit that brought together nearly two hundred experts, declared that they had discussed "several therapeutic and vaccine interventions that should be the focus of priority clinical evaluation at this time [and that] . . . a number of candidate vaccines and therapies have been developed and tested in animal models and some have demonstrated promising results. In view of the urgency of these outbreaks, the international community is mobilizing to find ways to accelerate the evaluation and use of these compounds."

Basically, it's about safety in humans versus possible adverse side effects. The current thinking is that the benefits of an effective vaccine outweigh the risk of side effects. When the safety issues are resolved, it is highly possible that the Ebola vaccine will become available relatively soon, first to health workers and then to the general public.

TIP

The WHO warns that you still need to remain cautious about the possibility of infection and not assume that a cure is forthcoming.

SHORT SUPPLY

In addition to the vaccines, the summit discussed the experimental drugs already available, though not in large enough quantities as of yet. As the statement explains, "Existing supplies of all experimental medicines are limited. While many efforts are underway to accelerate production, supplies will not be sufficient for several months to come. The prospects of having augmented supplies of vaccines rapidly look slightly better."

They also warn that ". . . investigation of these interventions should not detract attention from the implementation of effective clinical care, rigorous infection prevention, and control, careful contact tracing and follow-up, effective risk communication, and social mobilization, all of which are crucial for ending these outbreaks."

Although treatments and vaccines are under development, it still isn't likely that you can buy it at your local pharmacy anytime soon. The WHO warns that you still need to remain cautious about the possibility of infection and not assume that a cure is forthcoming.

OTHER COMPLICATIONS OF EBOLA

If Ebola proves fatal, death will occur within a week or two of the first symptoms, usually due to organ failure. If a patient survives Ebola, improvement will begin to show about two weeks after symptoms manifest.

If you are lucky enough to survive a bout with Ebola, you may still be faced with other complications for days, months, or longer. Due to its highly insidious nature, Ebola can take a toll on the body in many ways, including extreme weakness and fatigue, headaches, hair loss, chronic liver inflammation, sensory changes, and damage to certain organs. Hair and skin loss may occur as a possible result of infected sweat glands.

Also, the virus may yet persist for some infected through bodily fluids such as semen and breast milk—in some studies for up to three months. This means while the patient has been "cured," the disease can still be transmitted through sexual contact or breastfeeding months later. In 2000 in Uganda, two children died of Ebola after being breastfed by mothers who had recently recovered from the disease.

MORE HIGHLIGHTS FROM THE WHO SUMMIT

In September 2014 at a meeting of more than two hundred WHO leaders and Ebola experts, it was determined that the current Ebola epidemic is "the most severe acute public health emergency seen in modern times. Never before in recorded history has a biosafety level four pathogen infected so many people so quickly, over such a broad geographical area, for so long."

It was determined that there is a pressing need to "identify the most promising candidate vaccines and experimental therapies and map out the next most urgent steps to take. The experts agreed to prioritize convalescent blood and plasma therapies for further investigation." In reviewing the data, it was revealed that inroads had already been made in trying new therapies, aside from "supportive care," and the summit convened with a determination to get various treatments tested and approved as quickly as possible, stating that the "WHO has been encouraged by the growth of interest in convalescent therapies as an already bad epidemic gets worse."

The epidemic with world-changing implications is spurring researchers throughout the globe to find a way to treat and eradicate this terrible disease.

NOW YOU KNOW . . .
Ebola is diagnosed through a series of special tests. Right now, the way it is treated is through "supportive care," which means that the patient is supported by maintaining hydration and treating the symptoms as they appear. This is a strategy employed for many infectious diseases, even the common cold.

ZMapp is an experimental drug that has shown positive results in laboratory monkeys, and a few humans evacuated from the epidemic zone. While an effective Ebola vaccine may exist in the laboratory at the time of this writing, it is not yet widely available. Great strides are being made and it's possible that one will become available to the general public soon.

There's no certainty, however, so precautions still need to be taken. In the next part of the book, we'll discuss how to ensure you are and stay safe.

PART 2: PROTECTING YOURSELF AND YOUR FAMILY

For all there is to know about Ebola, the most important thing you need to concern yourself with is how NOT to get it. In this section, we'll look at measures you can take to keep yourself and your loved ones safe from this deadly disease.

5. Is Your Hospital Ready?

"ABOUT 70 HOSPITAL STAFFERS CARED FOR EBOLA PATIENT"

This headline from October 14, 2014, speaks specifically about Texas Health Presbyterian Hospital, the hospital in which Thomas Duncan received treatment for Ebola and died on October 6. One of the health-care workers, twenty-six-year-old Nina Pham, contracted Ebola, quickly followed by another, Amber Vinson. At the time of this writing, however, all the rest are still healthy.

There's been a lot of panic surrounding the infection of Nina Pham and Amber Vinson by Mr. Duncan, which is similar to the case of Madrid assistant nurse Teresa Romero. All of these incidents have been blamed on human error. CDC director Dr. Tom Frieden was in the forefront of those who blamed the new cases on "breaches of protocol."

A statement from the CDC went on that ". . . nurses, doctors, and other hospital employees wore face shields, double gowns, protective footwear, and even hazmat suits to avoid touching any of Duncan's bodily fluids." Therefore, they conclude that there had to have been a breach of protocol down the line.

"The first thing in caring for someone with Ebola is to do everything in your power to never become a victim," confirms Dr. Aileen Marty, a World Health Organization doctor. It would seem that somewhere down the line, an error had been made. I doubt that we will ever get confirmation of a specific mistake made. However, it is clear that our medical personnel are not getting the training, education, and protective gear needed to safely care for Ebola patients.

The group National Nurses United conducted an ongoing survey of 1,900 nurses. In the survey, 76 percent of all nurses indicated that they were unaware of any policy at their hospital on dealing with deadly epidemics. Eighty-five percent had no training sessions in which they could interact with an expert to ask questions. According to an Associated Press article on Mashable.com, gleaned from a statement by Deborah Burger of National Nurses United, Mr. Duncan:

> was left in an open area of a Dallas emergency room for hours, and the nurses treating him worked for days without proper protective gear and faced constantly changing protocols . . . Nurses were forced to use medical tape to secure openings in their flimsy garments, worried that their necks and heads were exposed as they cared for a patient with explosive diarrhea and projectile vomiting.

This seems like an inexcusable, even criminal negligence on the part of the hospital with regards to the safety of their nursing staff. Each day a new misstep was uncovered, each one worse than the last.

In response to the outcry of "sloppy" conditions at Texas Presbyterian, spokesperson Wendell Watson offered that: "Patient and employee safety is our greatest priority and we take compliance very seriously. We have numerous measures in place to provide a safe working environment, including mandatory annual training and a 24/7 hotline and other mechanisms that allow for anonymous reporting."

By the time the second health-care worker who treated Duncan at Texas Presbyterian, Amber Vinson, was diagnosed, the general public at large seemed convinced that the hospital

TIP

76 percent of all nurses indicated that they were un-aware of any policy at their hospital on dealing with deadly epidemics. Eighty-five percent had no training sessions in which they could interact with an expert to ask questions.

did not plan properly for Ebola patients. Not only that, but there was a deep sense of outrage when the news came out that nurse Vinson had been given the okay by the CDC to fly to Ohio after Mr. Duncan passed away, despite the fact that she had come down with a low-grade fever.

How could the CDC and the hospital have given such an authorization? If the call were made randomly to any average citizen, the answer would have been a resounding "no." It became clear that a clear national policy was deficient, if it existed at all. Indeed, the nation does not even have a Surgeon General at the time of this writing.

The human cost, in the lives of the two infected health workers, is immense. The financial cost, however, is almost as immense. The cost of treating Thomas Duncan during the time he was cared for at Texas Health Presbyterian Hospital has been calculated to be approximately $500,000 to one million dollars. That's one patient. Presumably this includes the cost of emptying out the entire ICU to care for the one Ebola case, but I'm not sure. Imagine the cost of 100 Ebola cases? 1,000?

How would you know if your hospital was safe should an outbreak occur around you? Read on.

DO WE HAVE THE TECHNOLOGY?

We like to think that Ebola spreads only in the Third World, where technology is not as sophisticated as in developed countries. Places like West Africa, where doctors are not specially trained and conditions are primitive. You might imagine slap-dash stretchers on dirt floors in "hospital rooms" that are really just canvas-covered tents. Well, it's not your imagination; it's the hard reality of life in the Ebola zone.

We know that there are less than ideal conditions in African countries where Ebola's spread has been rampant. The problems are huge there, but they also exist in the modern world. Texas Presbyterian Hospital and Madrid's Carlos III Hospital are large centers that are well financed. Yet for all their resources, they were equally as inadequate to safely deal with Ebola patients as the broken-down facilities in Liberia, Guinea, and Sierra Leone.

It's troubling, even frightening, to consider that your local hospital may be unsafe, especially if it has all the advances known and available to modern medicine. Even if it sets records for cleanliness and efficiency, it may still not be ready for an Ebola outbreak.

Does your hospital have a plan of action in place to deal with a serious epidemic? Has it given adequate training to its staff, and will it provide the protective gear necessary for them to safely treat contagious patients? These are good questions to ask your local hospital's administrator. If he or she answers "absolutely," I still wouldn't be convinced until they tell you how they reached that conclusion. If errors occurred at Texas Presbyterian, how is your local hospital any different?

I believe, in my heart, that the average hospital cannot handle the care of an Ebola or otherwise highly contagious patient. It's not their main job; they're used to medical problems like strokes, heart attacks, or injuries. There are very few hospitals that have the facilities and resources to ensure protection.

There are four high-risk infectious disease centers in the United States in Maryland (NIH), Atlanta (CDC), Nebraska, and Montana. I urge hospitals throughout the country to transfer all Ebola patients immediately to one of these centers. They are better equipped for the job.

WILL IT HAPPEN AGAIN?

In a recent article, CNN.com offered seven reasons why a situation that occurred in the Dallas hospital where Thomas Duncan died would never happen again. Here's the gist of what has been reported:

1. **Duncan wasn't hospitalized right away.** This was a result of the failure in the chain of communication. Texas Presbyterian will think again before sending home any patient with a fever and a West African travel history. Hospitals all over the nation will likely be more on guard about doing the same. A higher index of suspicion will lead to fewer discharges from emergency rooms until more testing is done.

2. **Duncan did not receive an experimental drug immediately.** The difference between the care of Dr. Kent Brantley, Nancy Writebol, and Dr. Richard Sacra, and that of Thomas Duncan, is that because Brantley and Writebol were quickly diagnosed with Ebola, they were given the experimental ZMapp drug early in the course

of the disease. Many attributed this to their successful recoveries (even though, honestly, we don't know). Hopefully, a stockpile of ZMapp may become available in the future.

3. **Duncan was given the wrong experimental drug.** When he was finally diagnosed with Ebola, he was given a drug called brincidofovir, a drug designed to inhibit the ability of the Ebola virus to replicate itself. While brincidofovir is already in Phase 3 clinical trials, it's not known whether it was not effective on Duncan because it simply didn't work, or if it was administered too late to save him. Once trials are completed, it will be clearer whether brincidofovir is effective or not.

4. **Duncan was not given a blood transfusion from an Ebola survivor.** In addition to giving infected patients ZMapp, it is suggested that blood or plasma transfusions from Ebola survivors may help combat the disease in victims. It is not known why Duncan was not provided this option; though, at the time of this writing, reports confirm that Nina Pham has been given a donation of plasma from Dr. Kent Brantley. Perhaps going forward, other hospitals will follow suit.

5. **Texas Presbyterian had no advance warning.** Emory knew exactly what was coming to them when Dr. Brantley and Nancy Writebol were delivered there direct from being infected in Liberia. Thomas Duncan was, in effect, the first walk-in. Yet, I disagree here. We were given warnings about Ebola. Its mere presence in an area easily reached by air travel should have been the warning. Our top health administrators failed to adequately plan ahead.

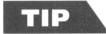

"Infections are a leading cause of deaths and complications for nursing home residents and, with the exception of tuberculosis, we found a significant increase in infection rates across the board."

Average citizens don't spend a great deal of time thinking about what they would do in an epidemic, and what the local health center would do to protect their health. They expect our appointed health officials to plan for them, and by doing so, ensure their safety.

INFECTIONS ARE RAMPANT

Hospitals and, especially, nursing homes are not always safe when it comes to infections. In fact, there have been documented cases of otherwise healthy people being admitted for various procedures and becoming sick. These illnesses are called hospital-based infections. It isn't the norm, but it's more common than anyone really wants to believe.

In a recent *Daily News* article, Carolyn Herzig, of the Columbia University School of Nursing, explained that "Infections are a leading cause of deaths and complications for nursing home residents and, with the exception of tuberculosis, we found a significant increase in infection rates across the board." Her team analyzed data submitted by nursing homes to the US Centers for Medicare and Medicaid Services between 2006 and 2010. They found rising rates of pneumonia, urinary tract infections, viral hepatitis, sepsis, wound infections, and multiple drug-resistant bacterial infections. Herzig believes, "Unless we can improve infection prevention and control in nursing homes, this problem is only going to get worse as the baby boomers age and people are able to live longer with increasingly complex, chronic diseases."

To a slightly lesser degree, this goes for hospitals as well.

Usually younger, otherwise healthy people do not get sick in hospitals. While anyone admitted to a hospital could contract a health-care-associated infection, some groups are definitely more at risk than others, such as the very young and the very old. Those with chronic medical conditions like diabetes and those with immune deficiencies are also at risk.

TAKING RESPONSIBILITY . . . OR NOT

Following Thomas Duncan's death, the CDC sent an alert to hospitals all over the country warning that: "Every hospital should ensure that it can detect a patient with Ebola." While a perfectly reasonable statement, it didn't outline a national policy for exactly how this should be accomplished. More importantly, it didn't mandate national guidelines for every hospital when it comes to staff education and training, protective gear requirements, and isolation room procedures. Even procedures as basic as how to put on and take off hazardous material suits are different based on the brand.

The issue with all of this is that hospitals are so decentralized that they are, apparently, not required to listen to the CDC. A spokesman for the National Nurses United union, Charles Idelson revealed that few hospitals have provided adequate education for their employees. Idelson says most are simply pointing nurses to information on their websites, or linking to CDC information.

One of the main issues with this is that despite the recent onslaught of coverage in the media over Ebola, it truly is seen as a third-world issue, and US hospitals are generally more inclined to put their resources into areas where they know for sure a condition exists because it's common to the population or the region. Think influenza in the wintertime in the Northeast.

Most hospitals already have systems in place for dealing with influenza outbreaks. They rely on these systems in the treatment of all highly contagious diseases, few if any of which have the death rate that Ebola has. As Dr. David Klocke, chief medical officer for Regional Health hospitals in South Dakota, explains, "We really are in general very well prepared to deal with dangerous microorganisms anyway."

Some might take the above statement as comforting, but I look at it and wonder if there's an aspect of arrogance in it. Is Dr. Klocke saying that his medical center can handle a community-wide Ebola outbreak? Given the circumstances, it would be a miracle if even the CDC could do so.

Going forward, we must do what can be done. Hospitals should be more vigilant about having nationally standardized practices in place for treating Ebola, and build a stockpile of materials that would make their efforts more successful.

WHOSE RESPONSIBILITY?

In the case of Texas Presbyterian, National Nurses United believes that procedures and protocols were definitely ignored or followed incorrectly. Although human error occurred, they feel that poor planning and mismanagement are the culprits that put the nurses who were infected at risk.

Management disagrees. A spokesperson for the hospital, Wendell Watson, made a statement that "Patient and employee safety is our greatest priority, and we take compliance very seriously" and that the hospital would "review and respond to any concerns raised by our nurses and all employees."

The Centers for Disease Control and Prevention stated that some breach of protocol probably sickened Nurses Pham and Vinson. National Nurse United claimed that protocols were either non-existent or were changed constantly after Thomas Duncan was admitted. Further investigation reveals other alarming allegations of protocol breaches, most by the hospital.

Ms. Pham was reportedly there from the beginning of his illness and treated Duncan throughout the course of his battle in the hospital's intensive care unit. Reportedly, "Duncan's medical records make numerous mentions of protective gear worn by hospital staff, and Pham herself notes wearing the gear in visits to Duncan's room. But there is no indication in the records of her first encounter with Duncan, on September 29, that Pham donned any protective gear."

How is that possible? How could Ebola not have been suspected as the cause of illness for a Liberian national who had traveled from Liberia shortly before ending up in that Texas emergency room?

According to National Nurses United, nurses from Texas Presbyterian have alleged that Duncan's "lab samples were allowed to travel through the hospital's pneumatic tubes, possibly risking contaminating of the specimen-delivery system [and] that hazardous waste was allowed to pile up to the ceiling."

TIP

There are no community-wide Ebola outbreaks here at present, and we can, under strong leadership, become capable of containing the disease in West Africa while protecting home territory. It will take a lot of humanitarian aid and tough, but logical, decision making.

It apparently wasn't for several days that protective gear, including shoe coverings, had been mandated for use in Duncan's care—that apparently there were a number of loose protocols and "recommendations" but very few essential hospital mandates.

Finally, several days into the ordeal, one of the nurses noted: "RN entered room in Tyvek suits, triple gloves, triple boots, and respirator cap in place." But what about all those days before? What kind of protections and precautions had been in place? The documentation is sparse.

It has been rumored that the staff at the hospital has been threatened with firings for speaking to the press, so it's hard to know if the public at large will ever know the real truth about how Duncan's care had been managed or mismanaged.

So who's at fault?

The medical staff may have committed errors in the donning and doffing of protective gear, if it was given to them in the first place. I have put on and taken off these outfits myself, and believe me when I tell you that there is a learning curve. A wrong move could easily mean contamination. Humans aren't perfect, and mistakes happen, but I believe in my heart that nurses are heroes and the heart and soul of the field of health care. I have seen what they do day in and day out, and I will admit to you, as a physician, that I couldn't do it.

The hospital has a burden of blame to bear, as it was clearly unprepared for dealing with the Ebola patient. It didn't have the equipment, the advanced training, and the policies in place that would have made the unit an effective team. To put it simply, the hospital was in over its head.

The blame falls, therefore, where the buck stops, and that's at the very top of our medical administration. Our top health officials have told us so often that we have nothing to worry about. We expect that we are up for any challenge because we are told that lie daily. I hoped that the high technology and vast resources in the United States would trump human error, disorganization, and yes, arrogance.

I was wrong. There are, indeed, circumstance for which we are unprepared, and woefully so. Our medical directors at the national level have failed to make us ready for the challenge of a deadly and contagious disease like Ebola. They have put considerations that may be political into an arena that should be apolitical. They have forgotten their duty to preserve the health of US citizens.

Yet, if any nation can rise to the challenge, we can. There are no community-wide Ebola outbreaks here at present, and we can, under strong leadership, become capable of containing the disease in West Africa while protecting home territory. It will take a lot of humanitarian aid and tough, but logical, decision making.

TAKING ACTION

To be fair, there has been some action on the part of the government. The CDC has sent a team to evaluate the systems in place at Texas Presbyterian to ensure the proper protocols are in place for the treatment of those affected as well as future cases. Among team members deployed to the hospital are experts in infection control, Ebola virus control and infectious diseases, laboratory science, personal protective equipment, hospital epidemiology, and workplace safety—and all members of the team have had specific experience with Ebola management, working with organizations including Doctors Without Borders.

Their investigation, which is pertinent to hospitals yet to have Ebola cases come in, has a number of focuses, including to evaluate how personal protective equipment (PPE) is being used and how it is being put on and taken off; what medical procedures were done on Mr. Duncan that may have exposed the health-care worker; the decontamination processes for workers leaving the isolation unit; ensuring oversight and monitoring of all infection control practices, particularly putting on and taking off PPE, at each shift in each location where this occurs should be implemented; and what enhanced training and/or changes in protocol may be needed.

From their evaluation of how things had been handled at Texas Presbyterian, by pinpointing what went wrong and how to correct it, the hope is that the team will be able to establish better, more specific guidelines for other hospitals to follow should an outbreak occur in other facilities.

HOSPITAL READINESS FOR A POSSIBLE
EBOLA OUTBREAK

There isn't a federal mandate on how Ebola should be handled; state and local guidelines still hold sway in these matters. The CDC reports: "Strict infection control is critical to stopping chains of transmission. Standard infection control practices in US health-care facilities apply to the safe management of patients with Ebola, but must be adhered to rigorously and meticulously. Hospitals should have staff practice the procedures and practice using the protective garb in advance."

But will hospitals follow the CDC's recommendations? This remains to be seen. The outbreak of Ebola in the United States is not considered an epidemic at the time of this writing. Therefore, many hospitals, as indicated above, are relying on the resources already in place for treating infectious diseases. Some hospitals may believe that an Ebola outbreak could never happen in the United States. This amounts to administrators and other professionals burying their proverbial heads in the sand.

However, some hospitals are beginning to see the wisdom in providing health-care professionals with additional training, plus education on the proper use and care of protective gear, including hazmat suits and masks.

One of the main reasons for the spread of Ebola in Sierra Leone and elsewhere is that while there may be protective gear available, it doesn't mean it's being used properly. The climate conditions in West Africa are oppressively hot and humid, with temperatures reaching 100 degrees Fahrenheit. Sometimes excessive condensation makes masks difficult to breathe through. It has been reported that workers can only handle being in full-body protective gear for just forty minutes before they become unbearably hot. Luckily, this

TIP

As Ebola is most commonly transmitted through direct contact with body fluids, or contact with contaminated objects, it's not as easy to contract Ebola as it would be to catch a cold, primarily transmitted through the air.

is not an issue in the hospitals in developed nations where the climate can be controlled, but there are other factors at work. Take, for example, a typical emergency room interview between doctor and patient. Essentially, it amounts to the ticking off of a checklist of symptoms; rarely is a travel history taken from an ER patient. The staffers, often with heavy patient loads, try and push through the waiting patients to decide if admittance to the hospital is necessary. In many cases, patients who are admitted must wait hours on a gurney before a bed becomes available.

Dr. Dino Rumoro, Rush UNI Medical Center's emergency medicine chief, says he's worked with worrisome diseases including AIDS, SARS, swine flu, and smallpox. As Ebola is most commonly transmitted through direct contact with body fluids, or contact with contaminated objects, it's not as easy to contract Ebola as it would be to catch a cold, primarily transmitted through the air. Rumoro has said, "At least with Ebola we have a fighting chance because I know that it is coming from body fluids and I know if I wear my (protective) suit I'm safe and I know if I don't stick myself with a needle or cut myself with a scalpel I'm safe."

The truth is that we are still uncertain about Ebola transmission, at least that's the opinion of the Center for Infectious

Disease Research and Policy (CIDRAP). Dr. Rumoro is correct that bodily fluids are the most likely mode of transmission, but we all must realize that there is a lot we still don't know about the disease.

There are more than 5,700 hospitals in the United States. However, CNN reports:

> That may seem like enough high-level centers that can handle Ebola safely, but there is one troubling statistic. There are only nineteen beds available total, if you add up all the beds in all four hospitals! The Nebraska Medical Center has the most beds, ten, while the others only have three each.

This is a real eye-opener and leads to the question: how can just four hospitals spread across the nation accommodate any significant outbreak of Ebola or, really, any truly dangerous infectious disease? They can't. That's why hospitals need to take measures to get themselves ready. Bruce Ribner, MD, medical director of the infectious disease unit at Emory University Hospital in Atlanta, stated, "It's not going to be possible, if this outbreak continues in West Africa, for a select number of institutions to care for patients."

The CDC has issued a preparedness checklist for hospitals to evaluate whether their current systems will be adequate to fight an Ebola epidemic should it ever arise at their facilities. If a patient in a US hospital is suspected or known to have Ebola virus disease, health-care teams should follow standard, contact, and droplet precautions, including the following basic recommendations:

- Isolate Ebola patients confirmed and suspected.
- Have health-care workers treat Ebola patients while wearing protective gear, including gloves, gowns (fluid

resistant or impermeable), eye protection (goggles or face shields), and facemasks, as well as double gloving, disposable shoe covers, and leg coverings.

- Do not permit visitors.
- Keep a log of everyone who comes in contact with the Ebola patient.
- Avoid aerosol-generating procedures wherever possible. (Did you know that flushing a toilet produces aerosols?).
- Implement environmental infection control measures by sterilizing non-disposable equipment and safely and carefully discard disposable hazardous waste.

As the old saying goes, "An ounce of prevention is worth a pound of cure." Hospitals may find their cases of Ebola can be controlled if they follow the CDC's recommendations and take proper precautions. Of course, there is always the possibility of human error, which means you need to be prepared beyond what hospitals may be able to offer.

NOW YOU KNOW . . .
Only four hospitals in the United States are fully equipped to handle and properly treat Ebola cases and only nineteen beds are available to treat all Ebola patients. While hospitals are upping their infectious diseases procedures and paying close attention to the particular demands of safe Ebola treatment, a great deal of improvement is needed. It's essential for you to make sure your local hospital has a workable plan to handle an Ebola outbreak should one occur in your area.

6. Common Sense Safeguards to Implement Now

With nineteen spaces in the four hospitals fully up to the task of treating Ebola patients, it's doubtful you will be admitted to one of these beds. Therefore, it makes logical sense that you want to do everything possible to prevent being infected. Liz Bennett wrote in *Underground Medic:*

> I think we just found out why the government(s) are underplaying the situation. They simply do not have the facilities to cope with even a small outbreak. They are, in fact in exactly the same position as the dirt-poor hospitals in West Africa . . . there are not enough facilities to stop the spread of the disease if it gets out.

If you think this is an alarmist statement, it's not. It's a reality. In this quick chapter, we'll look at some of the ways you can safeguard yourself and your family from Ebola.

For the first time in history, the UN is taking an Ebola outbreak seriously enough to institute safeguards against an international health crisis, warning that Ebola is "a threat to international peace and security." Anthony Banbury of the UN Security Council said in a statement that if the world did not meet critical goals by December, we would be facing ". . . an entirely unprecedented situation for which we don't have a plan." He goes on to explain that "Ebola got a head start on us, is far ahead of us, is running faster than us, and is winning the race" and that he is "deeply, deeply concerned" that an outbreak is imminent. The World Health Organization has stated that the response from developed nations has to increase twenty-fold to have a chance to contain the disease.

The safeguards recommended by the top hospitals and experts are:

- **Wash your hands!** One of the most important things you can do to prevent infectious disease is also the easiest – wash your hands frequently with soap and water. If you can't wash your hands, you can use alcohol-based hand rubs (like Purell), as long as they contain at least 60% alcohol. It's a good idea to keep hand sanitizer with you at all times, and use it after you shake hands or touch anything in a public place.
- **Stay away from infected people.** It's critical to especially avoid an infected person's bodily fluids, including blood, semen, vaginal secretions, vomit, and saliva. Ebola victims are most contagious when they are in the later stages of the disease and the virus is most plentiful in their bodies.
- **Wear protective clothing.** All health-care workers and caregivers should wear special protective clothing, including gloves, masks, gowns, and eye shields. Follow the CDC's latest recommendations for protective gear, and be sure to properly dispose of needles and other waste from the care of infected people.
- **Stay in safe areas.** Before traveling, make sure you're avoiding outbreak areas. You can check the most current epidemic information on the CDC website.
- **Do not go near dead bodies of victims.** The remains of Ebola victims can carry high quantities of the virus, so they should be handled by specially trained and equipped teams.

TIP

Wash your hands! One of the most important things you can do to prevent infectious disease is also the easiest— wash your hands frequently with soap and water.

BUT THAT'S NOT ALL . . .

The CDC adds to the list that you should:

- Avoid contact with bats and nonhuman primates as well as blood and other fluids from these animals.
- Avoid hospitals in West Africa where Ebola patients are being treated. The US embassy or consulate is often able to provide advice on safe facilities.
- After you return from any point of contact with Ebola, monitor your health for twenty-one days and seek medical care immediately if you develop symptoms of Ebola.

This is all helpful if you plan to travel to West Africa, but what should the average person in the United States do if he or she wants to prepare for a possible epidemic here? Later in this book, we'll talk about how to set up a sick room for infectious disease and what your strategy should be to keep your people healthy.

TAKING ACTION

Here are some examples of how areas in the United States and health-care systems have become more proactive since the current Ebola epidemic began.

In Brooklyn Park, which has a large Liberian population, police and firefighters will be taking additional precautions in light of the Ebola outbreak. They will wear eye shields and facemasks, as well as gloves, when responding to calls involving flu-like symptoms. They will also ask anyone with flu-like symptoms questions about any foreign travel. This includes not just the Liberians but the entire population of the city.

In New Jersey, all patients at Hackensack University Medical Center are screened for Ebola regardless of whether they've recently traveled to areas affected by Ebola, and the state reportedly provides regular Ebola health alerts to hospitals and other local health-care providers.

Dallas ambulance workers have become extra vigilant in cleaning and disinfecting ambulances after patient transport. An anti-microbial is sprayed on the stretcher, the straps, the rails, and anything else that might have been touched, and is left to soak for at least ten minutes before they wipe down the stretcher. "It's the universal precautions on steroids," said Dr. Frank Wright, the safety director of CareFlite ambulance service.

In Louisiana, the top education board has approved new school safeguards against the Ebola virus and other communicable diseases, including authorizing the closing of schools in the wake of a health crisis. Several Texas schools were closed when it was learned that some of their students were on the airplane with Ebola patient Amber Vinson.

Major airports now perform regular Ebola screenings on travelers from Liberia, Guinea, and Sierra Leone (more about this in the next chapter).

In addition, the nation's largest union of registered nurses has called on President Obama to mandate uniform standards at US hospitals to protect health-care workers from the Ebola virus.

EBOLA ACTIVISM

In addition to keeping yourself and your loved ones germ-free, you can take a larger role to spread knowledge about Ebola. Here are a few suggestions:

- Work to raise Ebola awareness in your area.
- Get support from your local politicians to help further awareness on the local, state, and national levels.
- Start a committee to establish guidelines for your local hospital to follow. Work with the hospital to get the systems in place.
- Donate money to a foundation (or create one) to help aid Ebola research and eradication. Recently, Facebook founder Mark Zuckerberg and his wife, Priscilla Chan, announced plans to donate $25 million to the Centers for Disease Control Foundation to help fight Ebola. Zuckerberg stated, "The Ebola epidemic is at a critical turning point. . . . It is spreading very quickly and projections suggest it could infect one million people or more over the next several months if not addressed. We need to get Ebola under control in the near term so that it doesn't spread further and become a long term global health crisis that we end up fighting for decades at a large scale, like HIV or polio."

Over the past decade, funding for initiatives like this has been cut dramatically. Dr. Francis Collins, the head of the National Institutes of Health, reports that "NIH has been working on Ebola vaccines since 2001. It's not like we suddenly woke up and thought, 'Oh my gosh, we should have something ready here.' Frankly, if we had not gone through our ten-year slide in research support, we probably would have had a vaccine in time for this that would've gone through clinical trials and would have been ready."

NIH's budget hasn't moved since 2004, when it was $28.03 billion—in 2013, it was $29.31 billion. Meanwhile, the National Institute of Allergy and Infectious Diseases' budget has fallen from $4.30 billion (2004) to $4.25 billion (2013). With inflation in account, that's a lot less money spent on protecting us from epidemic disease.

Instead, government has focused the CDC on other priorities, including community transformation. The CDC project on community transformation has received roughly three times the funding than the project to protect against infectious diseases. The program funds programs like "increasing access to healthy foods by supporting local farmers and developing neighborhood grocery stores" or "promoting improvements in sidewalks and street lighting to make it safe and easy for people to walk and ride bikes." Bike lanes and farmer's markets are laudable enterprises for any community, but they will do little to stem an outbreak of influenza, anthrax, or Ebola.

Don't think that I consider community transformation projects frivolous; for the most part, they're not. I believe, however, that they might be better funded by states, municipalities, or

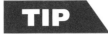

TIP

Over the past decade, funding for NIH initiatives have been cut dramatically. There is not much money being spent to protect us from epidemic disease.

private charities. Public health and safety is a better area for the federal government to spend resources. Let your local leadership know if this is how you feel.

EBOLA OPPORTUNISTS

In the wake of the Ebola crisis, plenty of predators are looking to capitalize on people's fears. Safeguarding is one thing; being played a fool and taken for a ride is a whole other story. Beware of people promising quick fixes and fail-safe protections from Ebola. Many of these have cropped up in recent months, including a purported Dr. Rima Laibow, who warns that Ebola amounts to a genocide and that she has something the public can buy to protect them.

About these so-called healers and their miracle cures, Better Business Bureau President Claire Rosenzweig says that the BBB and other agencies have received complaints about some natural products, such as a dietary supplement powder containing a fruit called garcinia cambogia, and an organic substance called monolaurin. Rosenzweig states, "They know that there's fear. They know there is anxiety." She adds, "All they're doing is getting you to catch the bait so they can hook you into buying their product."

With regards to protective gear, no affordable gear is fully safe when it comes to the advanced Ebola case. CIDRAP states that respirator masks (otherwise known as N95 masks) may be acceptable for the early stages of the disease. The complicating issue is that the quantity of virus in a late-stage patient may be so high that it penetrates the mask, which is designed to block 95 percent of particles above 0.5 microns in size (an N100 respirator masks blocks 99.7 percent, but is 15 times more costly). For advanced stages of the disease, a full hood with a powered air-purifying respirator (PAPR) is needed. These can cost $1,000 each, although some elements are reusable.

When you take into account all the items your outfit would include, it is prohibitively expensive to have all the personal protection equipment needed for care of the Ebola patient from first symptoms to recovery, especially when you consider that you might need to change several times a day. This consideration is a strong argument for my earlier assertion that Ebola patients must be transferred to high-level hospitals as soon as possible.

Having said all this, many items will give some protection and are worthy of consideration for handling various infectious disease issues. In the next chapter, we'll talk about these items and how they fit in your sick room supplies.

NOW YOU KNOW . . .
The best way to protect yourself and your loved ones against Ebola is to be proactive with preventative measures. Guidelines exist for travelers to West Africa from organizations involved

in containing the epidemic. In addition to washing your hands and using hand sanitizer, be careful where you travel and who you encounter.

Try to get involved in organizations working to prevent the spread of Ebola, and if none exist that fit the bill, consider starting one of your own. Donate money, if you can, to advance Ebola research or to send supplies to epidemic areas.

Above all, use your head. There are no quick cures when it comes to Ebola. Be skeptical if anyone promises you there are.

7. Safe Traveling

With commercial air travel, there just is no way that you're going to be able to contain anything or anyone anywhere for too long. The fact that it took Ebola nearly forty years to infect the United States is a pretty impressive example of successful containment.

Once here, it didn't take long for the virus to infect two health workers. The frustration here is those two cases would not have happened if there were travel restrictions from West Africa. Despite this, the government is not yet ready to consider this important option. Instead, they have instituted a screening process for travelers from the epidemic zone. According to the CDC, "Individuals who are determined to be at any potential risk will be actively monitored."

Humphrey Taylor, chairman of the Harris Poll, has said, "As the Ebola epidemic in West Africa continues to grow very rapidly, and the first American Ebola victims are being treated in this country, there is overwhelming support for strict screening of all new arrivals from the countries affected."

In fact, according to a recent poll, 58 percent of Americans would support a ban on incoming flights from Liberia, Guinea, and Sierra Leone. Another 22 percent couldn't decide if a travel ban would help matters or if proper screenings in airports might be enough. Only 20 percent believed a travel ban is a bad move. Despite this sentiment in support of travel restrictions from West Africa (not to), it's unlikely to ever happen.

Travel screening might be adequate, but only if the people screened are flying directly from countries that screen to the United States, without layovers in countries that don't screen Take the example of *NPR* producer Rebecca Hersher. She had a different story to tell when she traveled the same route Mr.

Duncan had taken. Hersher reported in detail, via tweets, all the information she was given in Liberia—all the times her temperature had been taken. After she transferred flights in Brussels, however, it was as though Ebola never existed until she landed back in the States and tweeted that once her passport was checked and it was noted that she had come from Liberia, she would be detained until a representative from the CDC spoke with her and evaluated her.

Brussels was the weak link. With little or no screening, potentially infected people from West Africa (or anywhere, really) could enter the country and depart right to the United States if they weren't visibly ill.

SHOULD TRAVEL TO AND FROM AFFECTED PARTS OF AFRICA BE BANNED?

Two sides of the argument exist. Hersher showed no signs of being sick, but why wasn't she evaluated more fully in Brussels? Gaps in screening on multiple-stop flights could miss someone with early symptoms.

Screenings expected to cover about 150 passengers per day are now in place in New York City's John F. Kennedy International Airport, Newark Liberty International Airport, Dulles International Airport outside Washington, DC, Chicago's O'Hare International Airport, and Hartsfield-Jackson International Airport in Atlanta. As previously mentioned, these are the five American airports that welcome 94 percent of travelers from Liberia, Sierre Leone, and Guinea into the United States. "It's not an effort that will be particularly disruptive to large numbers of people," CDC director Frieden explains. "We think

TIP

With the proper screenings, the experts believe that travel is safe, including travel to and from West Africa's Ebola-infected areas.

it is manageable." The CDC also plans to send additional staff to the five airports to support the new screening measures.

Many hope that screenings will suffice and that banning flights to and from stricken countries will not be the ultimate result. Director of Doctors Without Borders Christopher Stokes explains, "Airlines have shut down many flights, and the unintended consequence has been to slow and hamper the relief effort, paradoxically increasing the risk of this epidemic spreading across countries in West Africa first, then potentially elsewhere. We have to stop Ebola at [its] source and this means we have to be able to go there."

I have no disagreement with stopping Ebola at the source, but how are restricting travel *from* West Africa and sending relief efforts *to* West Africa mutually exclusive? They aren't. Some argue that restricting travel from the Ebola zone will damage the economies there. My response is that the economies are already in shambles in those nations, and that there is no reason to stop sending flights full of caregivers and medical supplies where they are needed. What is needed, however, is a way to prevent the importation of new Ebola cases.

Dr. Tom Frieden of the CDC refers to travel bans as "solutions that are quick, simple and wrong." Is the nation in agreement that it would be unfair to restrict West Africans from traveling to the United States? Twenty-two countries already do, including most African nations. In fact, Nigeria has successfully contained the epidemic with a travel ban, plus an incredibly stringent contact tracing program.

The concept of "fairness" relates to political correctness. The issue of travel restrictions should be as it is in other countries—a public health issue and not a political one. We cannot expect politicians to make the tough decisions between political correctness and public safety. Our top health officials are expected to do just that, however, and may have to before long to protect the health of US citizens.

IN THE MEANTIME . . .

With the proper screenings, the experts believe that travel is safe, including travel to and from West Africa's Ebola-infected areas. Essentially, anyone who travels to or from those areas will be given health information about Ebola and instructed in how to monitor themselves for symptoms.

Temperatures will be taken with specialized thermometers that do not make contact with their subject, and anyone with even a slight fever will be quarantined. There is no answer, however, to the question: What stops a person determined to get to the United States from taking acetaminophen (Tylenol) to keep their temperatures down artificially? Nothing.

If a passenger is directed to quarantine, the individual will be further examined for other symptoms of Ebola and either hospitalized or released. Dr. Frieden explains that health officials expect to see some patients with fevers during entry screening, "and that will cause some obvious and understandable concern at the airport," but people should not panic—thinking everyone who has a fever at the airport does not have Ebola.

Dr. Frieden is right when he says that most will have some other illness.

NOW YOU KNOW . . .
Better systems are now in place for screening international travelers for possible Ebola infection, but the system is not perfect and could possibly be circumvented. Travel restrictions from West Africa have become a political issue but should really be a public health issue. Any travel restrictions should leave an open door to relief flights to the affected countries of Liberia, Sierra Leone, and Guinea.

8. The Sick Room

The United States is lucky to have had few cases of Ebola on its shores, but who knows what will happen in the uncertain future. In good times, we have the luxury of modern medical facilities and advanced techniques to isolate a sick patient from healthy people. If we ever find ourselves in an epidemic scenario, hospitals will be overloaded and your only choice may be to fend for yourself. Our modern advantages will go the way of the dinosaur, and we will be placed in, essentially, the same medical environment we experienced in the nineteenth century.

Not completely, however. We have better knowledge of sterilization and the modes of transmission of infectious diseases like Ebola than we had in previous centuries. If we put this knowledge to work, the average person can become a medical asset in times of trouble.

With highly contagious diseases such as Ebola, it makes sense to separate the sick from the healthy. To do this, every household should designate a "sick room" before an epidemic arrives. The family "medic" can put together a working isolation area that will protect the healthy while giving an organized place to care for the sick.

When I say "protect the healthy," that means you as caregiver as well as everyone else. Ebola is harsh on medical personnel, infecting hundreds and killing more than half.

The sick room should be an area at one end of the house, preferably away from common areas like the kitchen. This room should have plenty of light and ventilation from the outside. Open windows will decrease the concentration of viral particles that may be suspended in the air. Assuming that you have power, air ducts are acceptable for diseases like Ebola, which is spread mostly via bodily fluids. For severe influenzas like bird flu, these ducts should be taped.

Your home may not be large enough to keep a clear space between the infected and the healthy. In this circumstance, screens and plastic sheets will come in handy. Even if the room has a door, plastic sheets should be hung to provide a barrier.

Furnishings in the sick room should be minimal. A bed or beds, an area for exams, a work surface, and a "latrine" may be sufficient for your purposes. Cloth surfaces, such as what you see in sofas, carpets, etc., can harbor pathogens (disease-causing organisms) and should be avoided, if possible. Plastic covers on bedding or furniture in the room will make daily cleanings more manageable. In the case of Ebola, a blood-splattered mattress may need to be thrown away and burned if it's not covered with plastic. Remember: the more areas that can be wiped down and disinfected easily, the better. Carpet and soft plush furnishings are your enemy.

It's important to have a way to eliminate waste products, especially from bedridden patients, even if it's just a five-gallon bucket and some bleach. Have closed containers like hampers to put used sick room items that need to be cleaned (or thrown away). We'll discuss proper disinfecting techniques later.

It's wise to establish a station near the entrance of the room or tent for masks, gloves, gowns, and disinfectants. Here you'll need a basin with water, alcohol, bleach, and towels that should be kept for exclusive use by the caregiver. If at all possible, there should only be one person involved in caring for an Ebola patient, in an effort to place few people at risk for contamination.

TIP

It's important to have a way to eliminate waste products, especially from bedridden patients, even if it's just a five-gallon bucket and some bleach. Have closed containers like hampers to put used sick room items that need to be cleaned (or thrown away).

The average citizen won't be able to afford $1,000 Powered Air-Purifying Respirator equipment. He or she will have to make do with items that will afford some protection, at least, from the infection.

For supplies, get plenty of masks and gloves. I strongly recommend putting on two pairs of gloves every time. Gowns can be commercially made, can be plastic coveralls, or, in extreme situations, even dry cleaner clothes covers. Many people consider medical supplies to consist of gauze, tourniquets, and battle dressings. These are useful for injuries, but you must also dedicate sets of sheets, towels, pillows, and other items to be used in the sick room. Keep these items separate from the bedding, bathing, and eating materials of the healthy members of your family or group. You'll never have enough of these items, as you'd discover if you found yourself having to deal with an Ebola victim.

Accumulating all these items may seem excessive to you, but you can never have enough dedicated medical supplies. You may save the life of a loved one or even your entire family if you are diligent in putting together your medical stores.

You'll want to clean the sick room as thoroughly as possible on a daily basis. It's imperative to clean surfaces that may have germs on them with a bleach-and-water solution. These include doorknobs, tables, sinks, toilets, counters, and even toys. Wash bed sheets and towels frequently; boil them if you have no other way to clean them. As a rule, all bedding, clothes, and personal items of the ill are infectious. Wash your hands right after touching them. The same goes for plates, cups, etc. Any equipment brought into the sick room should stay there.

You won't be able to give IV fluids to the Ebola patient in your sick room, but it's still important to keep them hydrated. They'll have many symptoms, like bleeding, that will be difficult to treat, but some medications will give "supportive care" to make them feel better and give their immune system an opportunity to kick in:

- Fever reducers (acetaminophen/Tylenol; stay away from ibuprofen or aspirin, as they could worsen bleeding issues)
- Pain relief (acetaminophen)
- Decongestants (pseudoephedrine/Sudafed)
- Antidiarrheals (loperamide/Imodium)
- Antinausea/vomiting drugs (ondansetron/Zofran)
- Vitamins and natural immune boosters
- Oral rehydration solutions
  These can be commercially purchased or you can make your own. To a liter of water, add:
    6–8 teaspoons sugar/liter
    1 teaspoon salt/liter (sodium chloride)

1/4–1/2 teaspoon salt substitute (potassium chloride)/liter

1/4 teaspoon baking soda/liter

For children, mix the above in two liters of water.

Give your patient a noisemaker of some sort that will allow them to alert you when they need help. This will decrease anxiety and give them confidence that you will know when they are in trouble.

Compare the above to official CDC recommendations for health-care professionals and you'll see that you can follow most of the guidelines in your own home rather effectively.

HEALTH-CARE PROFESSIONAL PRECAUTIONS

- Treat each person in their own area, with their own bathroom, if possible, or at least provide a barrier between patients.
- Take a careful log of medical professionals entering and exiting the room.
- Absolutely no visitors—only health-care providers permitted, and only those specially assigned to the case.
- Protective gear should be worn by all medical professionals entering the room—gloves, gowns (fluid resistant or impermeable), eye protection (goggles or face shields), facemasks, as well as double gloving, leg coverings, and disposable shoe coverings to protect from

copious amounts of blood, other bodily fluids, vomit, or feces present in the environment.

- Only dedicated, preferably disposable medical equipment is to be used. That which is not disposable needs to be cleaned and disinfected regularly.
- Limit use of needles, and take extreme care when used; dispose in puncture-proof, sealed containers.
- All aerosol-generating procedures should be avoided if possible; if not, a combination of measures to reduce exposures from aerosol-generating procedures should be employed, ideally in an Airborne Infection Isolation Room (AIIR) with closed door and limited exit and entry.
- Health-care providers should wear gloves, gowns, disposable shoe covers, and either a face shield that fully covers the front and sides of the face or goggles, and respiratory protection that is at least as protective as a NIOSH certified fit-tested N95 filtering face piece respirator or higher (e.g., powered air purifying respirator) during aerosol-generating procedures.
- The surfaces in the room should be cleaned regularly.
- Collection and handling of soiled reusable respirators must be done by trained individuals.
- Hands should be washed before and after all patient contact, and before putting on and upon removal of PPE, including gloves.
- If contact is made with fluids, health-care provider should stop working and immediately wash the affected skin surfaces with soap and water. Mucous membranes (e.g.,

TIP

Health-care providers should wear gloves, gowns, disposable shoe covers, and either a face shield that fully covers the front and sides of the face or goggles, and respiratory protection that is at least as protective as a NIOSH certified fit-tested N95 filtering face piece respirator or higher (e.g., powered air purifying respirator) during aerosol-generating procedures.

conjunctiva) should be irrigated with copious amounts of water or eyewash solution, and an occupational health/supervisor should be contacted for assessment.

- Health-care providers who develop sudden onset of fever, intense weakness or muscle pains, vomiting, diarrhea, or any signs of hemorrhage after an unprotected exposure (i.e., not wearing recommended PPE at the time of patient contact or through direct contact to blood or bodily fluids) to a patient with Ebola should immediately stop working, notify their supervisor, seek prompt medical evaluation and testing, notify local and state health departments, and comply with work exclusion until they are deemed no longer infectious to others.
- An asymptomatic health-care provider who had an unprotected exposure should receive medical evaluation and follow-up care including fever monitoring twice daily for twenty-one days after the last known exposure. (Source: CDC.gov)

DISINFECTANT SUPPLIES

Some supplies are disposable, but some aren't and can be reused. In good times, when items like coveralls are plentiful, these should be considered disposable. In a true pandemic setting, these supplies may be unavailable for the foreseeable future. In this case, you may have to make a decision to reuse supplies you should throw away. This is not something I think is wise, but your circumstances will dictate your actions. Understand that your level of protection will likely decrease significantly.

Disinfection, if done properly, will kill the Ebola virus. The virus is not particularly hardy, and simple materials like soap, alcohol, and bleach will help eliminate it from surfaces. Things that must be disinfected include:

- Hands and skin, whenever exposed
- Gloves
- Thermometers, stethoscopes, and other instruments
- Spills on walls, floors, or work surfaces
- Patient waste
- Patient bedding
- Needles and syringes

When disinfecting, use the same personal protection gear that you would when treating the patient.

BLEACH SOLUTION

A simple and inexpensive way to keep your sick room clean is with a solution of bleach. Ordinary household bleach can be prepared in a strong (1:10) solution and a weaker (1:100) solution. The strong version is for disinfecting patient waste and for disinfecting spills of blood, mucus, or other bodily fluids. The weaker version is useful for disinfecting surfaces, bedding, medical equipment, and reusable protective clothing (which shall then be washed). It can also disinfect aprons, boots, and items to be thrown away. Yes, items you discard must be disinfected.

To prepare a bleach solution, you'll need:

- A mixing container that can hold ten "measures." For example, a ten-cup container.
- Containers to hold the solutions (consider labels or separate colors for the 1:10 and 1:100 solutions).
- Chlorine bleach
- Clean water
- A measuring cup or similar item

Now, mark the mixing container at the 90 percent level. This will tell you the proper proportions for your mix. Then, pour water to the 90 percent level and add the rest with your bleach. You have just made your 1:10 solution.

To make your 1:100 bleach solution, pour water to the 90 percent level in a new container and use your 1:10 bleach solution to fill the rest of the way.

Prepare these solutions daily, as bleach loses its strength quickly. Smell the solutions; they should have a "bleach-y" odor. If they don't, the bleach has degraded and should not be used. For organization purposes, prepare your solutions at the same time every day.

CLEAN SURFACES

As surfaces such as tabletops, sinks, walls, and floors are not generally involved in the transmission of Ebola virus, they may not need intensive cleaning. However, daily maintenance is a good strategy.

WALLS, FLOORS, AND WORK SURFACES

For "clean" walls and floors, mop or otherwise clean with 1:100 bleach solution.

For spills or splatter on walls and floors, pour 1:10 bleach solution and let soak for 15 minutes before removing with a towel. Discard the towel.

BEDDING

For plastic sheeting: Remove liquid or solid waste with absorbent towels, then discard. Wash with 1:100 bleach solution daily.

For cloth sheeting: Remove sheets from the bed and place in a bucket or plastic bag. Soak in bleach solution for 30 minutes. Remove and place in soapy water overnight. Rinse and line-dry.

Mattresses: If heavily soiled, remove and burn (this is why plastic sheeting is so important). If the mattress must be reused, soak in 1:10 bleach until soaked on both sides. Dry in the sun (on both sides) for several days.

PATIENT UTENSILS

Eating utensils are medical supplies, too. Wash and rinse in 1:100 bleach solution and then air-dry.

PATIENT WASTE

Cover the contents of a bedpan or waste bucket with 1:10 bleach solution then empty the contents into a dedicated patient toilet or latrine. Rinse in 1:100 bleach solution before returning it to the sick room. For toilets, beware of splatter.

Burn towels, cloth, and paper waste after applying 1:100 bleach solution.

TIP

All instruments, such as stethoscopes or thermometers, should be washed after use. For this, you will use ordinary rubbing alcohol (70 percent isopropyl) or 1:100 bleach solution.

MEDICAL INSTRUMENTS

All instruments, such as stethoscopes or thermometers, should be washed after use. For this, you will use ordinary rubbing alcohol (70 percent isopropyl) or 1:100 bleach solution.

Place the alcohol or bleach in a container of appropriate size. This should be kept in the sick room. Dip a paper towel or clean cloth into it and wipe down the metal head of the stethoscope for 30 seconds. Glass thermometers may be soaked in the fluid for 10 minutes. Allow to air-dry and properly dispose of paper waste.

PROTECTIVE CLOTHING

Reusable clothing: Set aside a laundry area for Ebola patients. Place the laundry in 1:100 bleach solution and soak for 30 minutes, then place in soapy water. Soak overnight, then rinse and line-dry. Use worn clothing as cleaning implements.

Disposable clothing: Use 1:100 bleach solution then burn.

Boots: Have a pan with 1:100 bleach solution to clean soles and a sprayer for upper portions. Let air-dry.

Goggles: Dip in 1:100 bleach solution and air-dry.

Gloves: You should have these in quantity. Wear two pairs at a time. If there is more than one patient in the room, you could wash in soap and water and then dip in 1:100 bleach solution before going to the next patient. Dry first. The gloves won't last long using this method, so it is best to dispose after each use.

Masks: Dispose after each use.

ACCIDENTAL EXPOSURES

Many inexperienced or untrained medical personnel will have an inadvertent exposure on their skin to Ebola virus. This doesn't mean it's the end of the line. You can:

- Immerse the exposed area in rubbing alcohol for 20–30 seconds, then wash with soap and water.
- Flush the area with running water for 20–30 seconds
- If the skin has been broken, cover with a dressing.

NOW YOU KNOW . . .

A sick room should be designated to handle patients with infectious disease before an epidemic occurs. Furnishings should be minimal and utilitarian. Accumulation of medical supplies for the room should take into account bedding, utensils, protective clothing for caregivers, and disinfectants. Used items can sometimes be cleaned, but are best discarded in most cases. Bleach solution is effective in killing Ebola virus and is easily prepared, but must be replenished daily.

9. YOUR STRATEGY

Now you know how to create an effective sick room and how to keep it disinfected. At this stage, you should be accumulating supplies to furnish it and to disinfect items properly that will be used in the care of the Ebola patient.

Luckily, at the time of this writing, no community-wide outbreaks have ocurred in the United States. In the uncertain future, however, a true epidemic of Ebola or another infectious disease may arrive in your town. What should be your strategy in the event that multiple cases spring up in your area? What are some things you can do now to be ready?

The situation in Dallas should give you an indication of the level of vigilance that you should adopt. In Dallas, the only individuals to have contracted the disease from patient Thomas Duncan have been health-care workers who were in close proximity or handling his bodily fluids. So far, no casual contacts appear to have come down with the disease.

In this situation, the alert level for you, as an average person, is relatively low. You are unlikely to be involved in the care of an Ebola patient. No cases are turning up in the neighborhood. There are still hospitals with open beds, and efforts are being made to correct errors made in the care of the victims.

BEFORE THE YOU-KNOW-WHAT HITS THE FAN

What should you do right now to decrease your chances of catching infections and staying healthy? This applies to Ebola, but also goes for influenza or whatever the next epidemic candidate might be.

Wash your hands. Good hand hygiene will result in your being less likely to be infected with any infectious disease. When I say this, I mean washing your hands frequently. Over the course of a typical day, I'd like you to keep a running count of how many times you do this every day. Did you wash your hands every time you used a restroom? After you ate? After you shook hands with someone? After opening a door? Few people can say that they did. Certainly, this can amount to many hand washings a day.

The benefits of frequent hand washing (or using alcohol-based hand sanitizer) can hardly be denied. Concerned about getting dry hands? Use hand lotion. It may be an annoyance but it's much better than getting sick.

This is simple advice, but it isn't easy to get into the habit of frequent hand washing. Use common sense, and you'll realize how important it is to decrease the viral or bacterial count on your hands. Hand washing should be a developmental milestone for kids on the same level as toilet training.

Keep your hands off your face. Piece of cake, right? I doubt it. Observe one of your kids or friends for a half hour and count the times they touch their face with their hands. I'll bet you'd be surprised how often it happens. Each time is an opportunity for a disease-causing organism to get in your mouth, nose, or eyes.

Don't touch door handles with bare hands. After a trip to the restroom, use a paper towel, if available, to open the door as you leave. Bathroom door handles are loaded with germs. Throw the paper towel away as soon as you exit.

Boost your immune system. Eat healthily, avoid stress, get enough sleep, and stay fit. People who can accomplish these four things are in a lot better shape to resist infectious diseases.

Don't touch door handles with bare hands. After a trip to the restroom, use a paper towel, if available, to open the door as you leave. Bathroom door handles are loaded with germs. Throw the paper towel away as soon as you exit.

Some folks will take supplements of vitamin C, vitamin D, zinc, or selenium, all known to strengthen your immune system.

Make a plan of action. While things are still stable, figure out what you would do if you were in the midst of a full-blown epidemic. As previously mentioned, you should be mapping out that sick room. You should be accumulating supplies. If the going gets rough, you should be ready to get going.

THE EPIDEMIC ARRIVES

The going has just gotten rough. It's no longer just nurses and other health-care workers getting Ebola—it's the corner grocer, your neighbor down the street, and your buddy at work. The epidemic is ramping up into high gear, and you're smack dab in the middle of it. Your alert level is now HIGH. What do you do?

The strategy in this setting is known as "social distancing." Social distancing is a term applied to certain actions taken to stop or slow down the spread of a highly contagious disease. It's an important step to keeping your family healthy.

When there are people down the block who are sick, you know that the virus may be anywhere. The virus is still primarily transmitted by bodily fluids, so you don't necessarily have to hide behind a tree whenever you see another human being. You do, however, have to create a distance between yourself and the next person.

Avoid shaking hands with or hugging acquaintances. Stop receiving visitors at your home. Seriously consider whether your kids should go to school or whether you should go to that crowded office where you work. Poker night becomes a thing of the past. No political rallies or movie nights. Many people in Asia socially distance themselves when sick or when an epidemic is raging in the area. You've probably seen images of an Asian city street with a number of people wearing masks. It may appear silly to you, but it's a sign of social responsibility to them, and they're right. You never know which contact could pass the virus to you and then to your family.

At this point, you'll take out those items for your sick room and get it equipped. When someone is sick with Ebola, they could easily collapse in your kitchen. You don't want them in your common areas, but there they'll stay until you have the sick room with the plastic sheeting up and running. If someone becomes ill, you can transport them straight to the sick room if you already have it set up.

Stock up. While the stores still have food, get enough to last you a good long while. Concentrate on nonperishables and stockpile water supplies. Get equipment that would allow you to make fires for cooking and disposing of hazardous waste. If your area gets quarantined, you might have to depend on what you have on hand.

Other helpful items to have on hand include:

- Firestarters, candles, matches, lighters
- Propane fuel for cooking
- Flashlight or other light source and batteries

- Hand-crank radio
- Axe and knife
- First aid kit

Hit the road, Jack. There may come a time when your healthy family is surrounded by victims of the epidemic. You might just have a vacation home in a remote area or a favorite camping spot that no one else knows about. This is a serious decision, but it may be an option in dire times.

While you can still get fuel, keep your vehicle's gas tank filled to the top. You can get a good distance away if you have a place to go. Prepare "go bags" packed with changes of clothes, toiletries, and individually packaged nonperishable food and bottles of water in case evacuation becomes imminent.

If you're heading for the woods, you'll need a tent, sleeping bags, tarps, and other necessities for a reasonable shelter. Outdoor clothing and a good set of boots are a must, as well. A good compass is never a bad idea, as well as whistles for everyone in case you get separated.

NOW YOU KNOW . . .
Frequent hand washing is the best way to avoid getting sick from many infectious diseases, including Ebola. Keep your hands off your face to decrease the risk of disease. Planning a sick room will keep you prepared if an epidemic breaks out in your area. Social distancing is a strategy that will decrease your number of contacts and your chance of contracting contagious diseases. Having stockpiles of food, water, gas, and other items will keep you going if everything else fails. Tough decisions, such as whether to stay where you are or risk travel to other areas, are part and parcel of epidemic scenarios.

10. Worldwide Pandemic

Suzanne Hamner wrote on *Freedom Outpost* that "our government failed to protect the citizenry from the outbreak of this dangerous, deadly, contagious [disease] by suspending air travel to and from suspected areas or securing our southern border. At a time when communities deserve truth instead of over-confidence, our government has insured over-confidence is to be the face of the health-care community."

Indeed, we have been told so often that "all is well" that the average person has become either oblivious or extremely suspicious that all is *not* well.

While a work of fiction, Stephen King's *The Stand* showed all too well how one careless act involving infectious material can lead to a nearly worldwide annihilation of humanity. *The Stand* is one of my favorite books from years before I ever became interested in medical preparedness. Clearly, the Ebola virus is a perfect analogy for the "Superflu" described in the book. It's deadly, it's contagious, and it can turn society on its ear if not contained.

EBOLA AS A BIOLOGICAL WEAPON

Given my fondness for Stephen King's *The Stand*, you would think that I would be a big conspiracy theorist or someone who strongly suspects that Ebola has been unleashed purposefully on an unknowing and ill-prepared world. I'm not. That doesn't mean I would be surprised if Ebola virus samples turned up in some country's secret laboratory, but it does mean that I can critically evaluate whether it is really that amenable to weaponization.

As I discuss on my website, biological warfare is the use of infectious agents such as bacteria, viruses, fungi, or their by-products to wreak death and havoc among a specific population. The user's goal is to achieve control over an area or a segment of the population by weakening the ability to resist. Biological weapons don't necessarily have to kill directly: unleashing a horde of locusts to destroy crops or agents that kill an area's livestock can be just as effective.

The perfect biological weapon would have these characteristics:

- Be infectious and contagious in a large percentage of those exposed
- Cause severe long-term debilitation or death of the infected organism
- Have few available antidotes, preventives, or cures
- Be easily deliverable to the area or population targeted
- Have low likelihood of causing damage to those using the agent

From my research, Ebola virus doesn't make the grade. Ebola virus is very sensitive to its environment and just doesn't last long outside a host. It doesn't tolerate sunlight and needs high temperature and humidity to survive. Most cities in developed countries don't have the climate conducive to Ebola's survival.

Viruses live in hosts, and with commercial air travel, I would guess that it's possible that an Ebola patient in Texas or Florida could travel with the virus to North Dakota or Minnesota. The fact is, however, that no epidemic outbreak of Ebola has ever spontaneously occurred outside of a hot, humid region.

TIP

Most cities in developed countries don't have the climate conducive to Ebola's survival.

Ebola is also not easy to work with. Even if a terrorist kidnapped an Ebola victim to get viral samples, working with the virus in anything less than an advanced microbiology lab (called a "Biosafety Level 4") would likely result in the terrorist dying from the disease. As well, Ebola virus is too sensitive to survive the complex process of refining, enriching, and so on that is necessary for weaponization.

So don't panic the next time you read about "Ebola Gas" or "Ebola Bombs." Be aware of the virus, have supplies available that will help in a crisis, and use your most important survival tool: your mind. Do your research and get the facts to come to a conclusion.

THE BOTTOM LINE

Government and health officials will continue to downplay the notion that Ebola could reach apocalyptic proportions to avoid wholesale panic, even if four thousand American military personnel are deployed to the epidemic zone. To be prepared, however, it's important to always stay aware of the facts and never assume that it couldn't happen here.

Americans need to prepare by making a plan of action that can be activated if Ebola ever reaches their area. They must also continue asking the tough questions of those in power.

The American Thinker blog offers fourteen questions that will never be asked about Ebola but should be. They include:

- "Why doesn't the United States have a mandatory quarantine period of twenty-eight days before allowing any traveler who has visited West Africa in the past ninety days, to enter our country?"
- "If an outbreak of Ebola occurs in a major US city such as New York, Chicago, or Los Angeles, is this government prepared to quarantine five to eight million citizens from land, sea, and air travel to stop the spread of the virus? How many deaths from such an outbreak would trigger such quarantine? Would US troops be ordered to fire upon US citizens attempting to evade the quarantine?"
- "How many Ebola deaths nationally would trigger a Presidential Executive Order declaring martial law, nationalizing the distribution of food, energy, health care, and information? Would this Executive Order also limit the duration of martial law and the circumstances for it being lifted?"

And, perhaps most significantly:

- "Why are so few of us raising our voices—screaming at the top of our lungs—demanding that our government begin implementing common-sense epidemiological safeguards against Ebola unnecessarily infecting more Americans?"

The United States, more than any other country, has the potential to rise to the challenge of containing this epidemic and helping those in need. We must expand our efforts in West Africa and remain the force of good for the world that we have traditionally been.

By the same token, the United States can't ignore the public health and safety of its citizens. Americans depend on government to protect the populace in times of trouble. We have to look at the Ebola crisis in terms of humanitarian considerations, but also in terms of self-preservation. That means that there may be tough decisions ahead.

I hope that the reader of this book never has to resort to the strategies that I've outlined here. I prefer to hope for the best, while preparing for the worst. In this way, we can all succeed, even if everything else fails.

NOW YOU KNOW . . .
A heckuva lot about Ebola. I hope that, for your family, it will be, in the distant future, just a number of interesting facts you learned a long time ago.

RESOURCES

The Center for Disease Control and Prevention
http://www.cdc.gov/

The World Health Organization
http://www.who.int/en/

The National Institutes of Health
http://www.nih.gov/

The American Medical Association
http://www.ama-assn.org/ama

The New England Journal of Medicine
http://www.nejm.org/

The American Red Cross
http://www.redcross.org/

Doctors Without Borders
http://www.doctorswithoutborders.org/

US Department of Health and Human Services Disaster Information Management Resource Center
http://sis.nlm.nih.gov/dimrc/Ebola_2014.html

Mayo Clinic
http://www.mayoclinic.org/

ALSO AVAILABLE

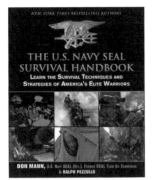

The U.S. NAVY SEAL SURVIVAL HANDBOOK
Learn the Survival Techniques and Strategies of America's Elite Warriors

Don Mann
Ralph Pezzullot

The U.S. Navy SEAL Survival Handbook, from decorated Navy SEAL Team Six member Don Mann, provides a definitive survival resource.

$17.95 Paperback
978-1-61608-580-3

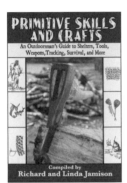

Primitive Skills and Crafts
An Outdoorsman's Guide to Shelters, Tools, Weapons, Tracking, Survival, and More

Linda and Richard Jamison

Anyone eager to master survival skills for outdoor vacations, or simply to find a fun new family activity for a Saturday afternoon, will be educated and inspired by the practical advice presented here by archaeologists, anthropologists, primitive practitioners, craftsmen, and artisans.

$12.95 Paperback
978-1-60239-148-2

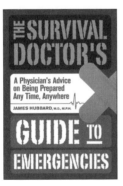

The Survival Doctor's Guide to Emergencies
A Physician's Advice on Being Prepared Anytime, Anywhere

James Hubbard

The Survival Doctor's Guide to Emergencies teaches lay people step-by-step essentials to medical care during a crisis. Most of us want to be self-reliant and in control of our fate as much as possible.

$16.99 Paperback
978-1-63220-716-6

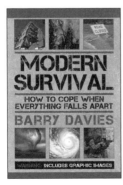

Modern Survival
How to Cope When Everything Falls Apart

Barry Davies

Tornadoes, floods, and terrorism—frightening events like these are in the news every day. Davies, a British Special Air Service veteran, will help you prepare so that you're not only able to survive but are also able to continue on with your life healthily and successfully once the dust has settled.

$16.95 Paperback
978-1-61608-552-0

ALSO AVAILABLE

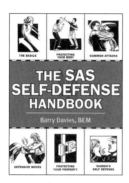

The SAS Self-Defense Handbook
Barry Davies

Barry Davies is one of the most widely respected experts on the techniques and training of the elite British Special Air Service (SAS). The handbook is fully illustrated with nearly 130 photographs and illustrations that explain how to properly use your body and use everyday objects such as desktop items and cigarette lighters to protect yourself.

$12.95 Paperback
978-1-61608-290-1

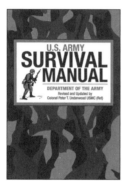

U.S. Army Survival Manual
Department of the Army
Revised and updated by Peter T. Underwood

Whether you're gearing up for a backcountry trek, preparing for the worst that nature or man can offer, or just want to have a great resource at your fingertips, you need this comprehensive, full-color new edition of the *U.S. Army Survival Manual*, thoroughly revised by Colonel Peter T. Underwood, USMC (Ret.).

$12.95 Paperback
978-1-62636-158-4

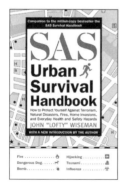

SAS Urban Survival Handbook
How to Protect Yourself Against Terrorism, Natural Disasters, Fires, Home Invasions, and Everyday Health and Safety Hazards

John "Lofty" Wiseman

We are constantly reminded that the world is a dangerous place. Wiseman shows readers how to think realistically and practically about these perils in order to avoid them, whether they are at home, on the street, in school, or in transit.

$17.95 Paperback
978-1-62087-711-1

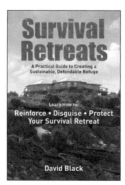

Survival Retreats
A Practical Guide to Creating a Sustainable, Defendable Refuge

David Black

In *Survival Retreats* you'll learn how to protect and defend your retreat, where to build it, and tips for living in your retreat. Black goes into detail to teach you everything you ever needed to know about survival retreats.

$14.95 Paperback
978-1-61608-417-2

ALSO AVAILABLE

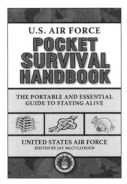

U.S. Air Force Pocket Survival Handbook
The Portable and Essential Guide to Staying Alive

United States Air Force
Edited by Jay McCullough

This new edition will allow you to carry formal Air Force training information condensed in your back pocket. For the general reader, it offers a complete and comprehensive manual of outdoor survival techniques.

$12.95 Paperback
978-1-62087-104-1

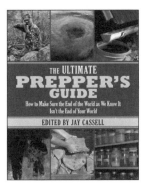

Bushcraft
The Ultimate Guide to Survival in the Wilderness

Richard Graves

Many have died in the Australian bush who might have lived had they known the appropriate survival skills. *Bushcraft* covers all areas of survival and camping activities: making ropes and cords, building huts, camp craft, finding food and water, making maps, starting fires, tying knots, and fashioning hunting and trapping gear.

$16.95 Paperback
978-1-62087-361-8

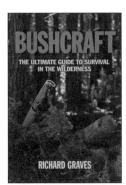

The Ultimate Prepper's Guide
How to Make Sure the End of the World as We Know It Isn't the End of Your World

Edited by Jay Cassell

The Ultimate Prepper's Guide is packed with practical approaches, step-by-step instructions, and how-to explanations for disaster and emergency preparation. Knowledge maps, flow charts, and templates provide important information at a glance and walk you through your decisions on personalizing and customizing disaster preparation.

$24.95 Paperback
978-1-62873-705-9

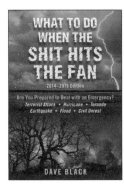

What to Do When the Shit Hits the Fan
2014-2015 Edition

Dave Black

Recent events have taught us all that anyone, anywhere can face an emergency situation. Do you have the tools, equipment, and knowledge to ensure the safety of your family? With the expert advice in this handbook, you can be better prepared for any emergency.

$12.95 Paperback
978-1-62636-109-6

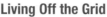

ALSO AVAILABLE

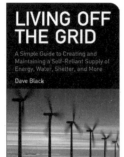

Living Off the Grid
A Simple Guide to Creating and Maintaining a Self-Reliant Supply of Energy, Water, Shelter, and More

Dave Black

Dave Black describes alternatives for eco-pimping your home and lifestyle for independence, economy, and a more integrated way of life. Equally valuable for the urban dweller vaguely concerned about the size of his or her carbon footprint and the rural self-sufficiency enthusiast

$12.95 Paperback
978-1-60239-316-5

52 Prepper Projects
A Project a Week to Help You Prepare for the Unpredictable

David Nash
Introduction by James Talmage "Dr. Prepper" Stevens

Are you and your family self-reliant? Will you be able to provide for them and keep them safe? The best way to prepare for the future is not through fancy tools and gadgets—it's experience and knowledge that will best equip you to handle the unexpected.

$16.95 Paperback
978-1-61608-849-1

52 Canning and Preserving Techniques for Preppers
A Strategy a Week to Help Stock Your Pantry for Survival

David Nash

In *52 Canning and Preserving Techniques for Preppers*, you'll find a project for every week of the year, designed to teach you the fundamentals of canning and preserving any sort of food as safely as possible. It doesn't matter how prepared you are for disaster, if you run out of food you will soon run out of time.

$16.99 Paperback
978-1-63220-634-3

The Prepper's Pocket Companion
How to Prepare for the End of the World as We Know It

Kate Rowinski

The Prepper's Pocket Companion shows you what to do before, during, and after any disaster, whether big or small. A cataclysm can happen in an instant and without warning, and you won't be able to save yourself if you are not prepared.

$14.95 Paperback
978-1-62087-261-1

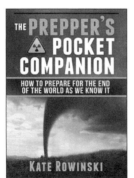